Telemedicine

Editor

AARON J. SMILEY

VETERINARY CLINICS OF NORTH AMERICA: SMALL ANIMAL PRACTICE

www.vetsmall.theclinics.com

September 2022 • Volume 52 • Number 5

ELSEVIER

1600 John F. Kennedy Boulevard • Suite 1800 • Philadelphia, Pennsylvania, 19103-2899
http://www.vetsmall.theclinics.com

**VETERINARY CLINICS OF NORTH AMERICA: SMALL ANIMAL PRACTICE Volume 52, Number 5
September 2022 ISSN 0195-5616, ISBN-13: 978-0-323-96159-2**

Editor: Stacy Eastman
Developmental Editor: Axell Ivan Jade Purificacion

Veterinary Clinics of North America: Small Animal Practice (ISSN 0195-5616) is published bimonthly by Elsevier Inc., 360 Park Avenue South, New York, NY 10010-1710. Months of issue are January, March, May, July, September, and November. Business and Editorial Offices: 1600 John F. Kennedy Blvd., Ste. 1800, Philadelphia, PA 19103-2899. Customer Service Office: 3251 Riverport Lane, Maryland Heights, MO 63043. Periodicals postage paid at New York, NY and additional mailing offices. Subscription prices are $369.00 per year (domestic individuals), $980.00 per year (domestic institutions), $100.00 per year (domestic students/residents), $465.00 per year (Canadian individuals), $1029.00 per year (Canadian institutions), $503.00 per year (international individuals), $1029.00 per year (international institutions), $100.00 per year (Canadian students/residents), and $220.00 per year (international students/residents). To receive student/resident rate, orders must be accompanied by name of affiliated institution, date of term, and the *signature* of program/residency coordinator on institution letterhead. Orders will be billed at individual rate until proof of status is received. Foreign air speed delivery is included in all *Clinics* subscription prices. All prices are subject to change without notice. **POSTMASTER:** Send address changes to *Veterinary Clinics of North America: Small Animal Practice*, Elsevier Health Sciences Division, Subscription Customer Service, 3251 Riverport Lane, Maryland Heights, MO 63043. Customer Service (orders, claims, online, change of address): Elsevier Periodicals Customer Service, Elsevier Health Sciences Division Subscription **Customer Service 3251 Riverport Lane Maryland Heights, MO 63043. Tel: 1-800-654-2452 (U.S. and Canada); 314-447-8871 (outside U.S. and Canada). Fax: 314-447-8029. E-mail: journalscustomerservice-usa@elsevier.com (for print support); journalsonlinesupport-usa@elsevier.com (for online support).**

Reprints. For copies of 100 or more of articles in this publication, please contact the Commercial Reprints Department, Elsevier Inc., 360 Park Avenue South, New York, NY 10010-1710. Tel.: 212-633-3874; Fax: 212-633-3820; E-mail: reprints@elsevier.com.

Veterinary Clinics of North America: Small Animal Practice is also published in Japanese by Inter Zoo Publishing Co., Ltd., Aoyama Crystal-Bldg 5F, 3-5-12 Kitaaoyama, Minato-ku, Tokyo 107-0061, Japan.

Veterinary Clinics of North America: Small Animal Practice is covered in *Current Contents/Agriculture, Biology and Environmental Sciences, Science Citation Index, ASCA, MEDLINE/PubMed (Index Medicus), Excerpta Medica,* and *BIOSIS.*

Contributors

EDITOR

AARON J. SMILEY, DVM
Chief of Staff Advisor, VetCor, Hingham, Massachusetts; Chief of Staff, Devonshire Veterinary Clinic, Anderson, Indiana; Veterinarian, Medici, Austin, Texas

AUTHORS

SHEA COX, DVM, CVPP, CHPV, RN
BluePearl Pet Hospice, Blue Pearl Specialty and Emergency Pet Hospital

MARK CUSHING, JD
Founder and CEO of Animal Policy Group, Scottsdale, Arizona

KATHERINE DONAHUE, DVM
Veterinary Medical Director, GuardianVets, Chicago, Illinois

DYLAN JONES, MS
Texas Christian University, United States Air Force, Veteran, President, Animal Cloud Device Connectivity, Inc

TIMOTHY MANZI, VMD
Diplomate, American College of Veterinary Radiology; Diplomate, American College of Veterinary Radiology - Equine Diagnostic Imaging; University of Pennsylvania, Clinical Studies New Bolton Center, Kennett Square, Pennsylvania

ASHLEY MITEK, DVM, MS
Diplomate, American College of Veterinary Anesthesia and Analgesia; Owner, AnesthesiaDiva.com, Co-Founder, Startocyte.com, Department of Veterinary Clinical Medicine, Teaching Assistant Professor, University of Illinois College of Veterinary Medicine, CEO & Co-Founder, Stratocyte, Urbana, Illinois

CRISTOBAL NAVAS DE SOLIS, LV, PhD
Diplomate, American College of Veterinary Internal Medicine (Large Animal); University of Pennsylvania, Clinical Studies New Bolton Center, Kennett Square, Pennsylvania

ANDREW NEWELL, BSBA
Vice President, Animal Cloud Device Connectivity, Inc; University of Colorado, Boulder, Colorado

AARON J. SMILEY, DVM
Chief of Staff Advisor, VetCor, Hingham, Massachusetts; Chief of Staff, Devonshire Veterinary Clinic, Anderson, Indiana; Veterinarian, Medici, Austin, Texas

SAMANTHA VITALE, DVM, MS
Diplomate, American College of Veterinary Internal Medicine (Neurology); President, Stratocyte

Contents

Preface: Veterinary Remote Care

Aaron J. Smiley

ix

What Is Telemedicine, Telehealth, and Teletriage

Mark Cushing

1069

In this article, the author reviews a history and overview of veterinary telemedicine and telehealth and human health heritage. Definitions and best practices for veterinary telemedicine and telehealth include key distinctions between the two.

Teletriage-How Remote Advice Provides Better Care

Katherine Donahue

1081

There are veterinary deserts across the country where access to veterinary care is limited. Teletriage allows animal owners in these areas to get expert advice about the time frame for care through convenient, commonly used methods of communication. Teletriage also creates financial benefits for traditional veterinary clinics by increasing scheduling efficiencies. Lastly, teletriage can creates employment opportunities for veterinary nurses without the burden of relocation.

Wearable Devices in Veterinary Health Care

Ashley Mitek, Dylan Jones, Andrew Newell, and Samantha Vitale

1087

Wearables are an up-and-coming tool in veterinary health care. This article reviews the current and prospective wearable technology for veterinary patients and the future of wearables in veterinary medicine. These devices allow veterinarians to monitor a patient's vital signs remotely, in addition to other variables, and push the profession away from a reactive health-care system toward a proactive culture that is able to identify diseases earlier. Advances in this technology have the potential to profoundly change the way veterinarians obtain and use patient data to practice medicine.

Anesthesiologists in the Ether: Technology and Telemedicine in Anesthesiology

Ashley Mitek

1099

A new frontier in veterinary anesthesia telehealth has begun. With the adoption of electronic anesthetic records and video, phone, and chat consultations, an anesthesiologist can be integrated into the care team of any patient, anywhere in the world. This article reviews the benefits of adopting an electronic anesthetic record system, and the ways that practitioners can incorporate a virtual anesthesiologist into their care team.

Technology Basics for Telemedicine: What Practitioners Need to Know   1109

Ashley Mitek

Veterinary medical technology is rapidly evolving and provides exciting opportunities for veterinarians to practice medicine in new ways. This article reviews the basic components of telemedicine technology that practitioners should be aware of.

Telehealth in Hospice and Palliative Care   1123

Shea Cox

Hospice and palliative care is a framework of care focused on the palliation of a patient's pain and symptoms while attending to the emotional and spiritual needs of the client caregiver. Telehospice and telepalliative care is the use of telehealth services for delivering hospice and palliative care to patients remotely through videoconferencing, telephonic communication, or remote symptom monitoring and can address the needs of both patients and clients. Telehealth-based interventions can provide hospice and palliative care providers the ability to assess and address patient care needs including the delivery of effective pain and symptom management, timelier assessments and medical interventions, increased compliance, and additional teaching opportunities for clients.

Asynchronous Veterinary Telemedicine   1135

Aaron J. Smiley

Asynchronous communication is the predominate modality for present day communication. Veterinarians can become more efficient and create more access to care if they incorporate more asynchronous care into daily practice. This article reviews how veterinary medicine has used asynchronous communication in the past, the advantages of asynchronous telemedicine, and the inclusion of the client in virtual referral.

Small Animal Teleultrasound   1141

Timothy Manzi and Cristobal Navas de Solis

Teleradiology is well established in many small animal practices, whereas teleultrasound is slowly gaining prominence. The demand for teleultrasound services in the veterinary profession has increased substantially because access to ultrasound to general practitioners increases faster than the number of imaging specialists and Point of Care Ultrasound (POCUS) becomes part of the standard of care. Two main methods of teleultrasound currently exist: asynchronous (eg, "store-and-forward") and synchronous (eg, real-time) interpretations. Few standardized protocols for teleultrasound in small animals are available. Similarly, there are no standardized training programs for sonographic examination acquisition and interpretation outside of the traditional diagnostic imaging residency under the purview of the American College of Veterinary Radiology. The success of a telesonographic evaluation largely depends on the relationship between the veterinarian requesting remote assistance and the expert providing support.

VETERINARY CLINICS OF NORTH AMERICA: SMALL ANIMAL PRACTICE

FORTHCOMING ISSUES

November 2022
Vector-Borne Diseases
Linda Kidd, *Editor*

January 2023
Clinical Pathology
Maxey L. Wellman and M. Judith Radin, *Editors*

March 2023
Ophthalmology in Small Animal Care
Bruce Grahn, *Editor*

RECENT ISSUES

July 2022
Small Animal Orthopedic Medicine
Felix Duerr and Lindsay Elam, *Editors*

May 2022
Hot Topics in Small Animal Medicine
Lisa L. Powell, *Editor*

March 2022
Soft Tissue Surgery
Nicole J. Buote, *Editor*

SERIES OF RELATED INTEREST

Veterinary Clinics: Exotic Animal Practice
https://www.vetexotic.theclinics.com/

THE CLINICS ARE NOW AVAILABLE ONLINE!
Access your subscription at:
www.theclinics.com

Preface
Veterinary Remote Care

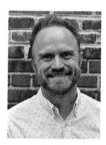

Aaron J. Smiley, DVM
Editor

It is my hope that the articles in this issue reveal the longstanding tradition of telemedicine in the veterinary profession and the skill veterinarians possess to care for their patients remotely. Veterinary telemedicine has persisted for over 150 years and is now rapidly expanding because technology allows the veterinarian to directly evaluate the patient in an ever-increasing number of ways. Telemedicine technology does not supplant the veterinarian. It gives the doctor additional tools to provide better care to more patients.

I am grateful for the time and expertise each author sacrificed to create his article, and I am honored to edit this issue. I am hopeful that the information in this issue generates ideas that materialize into technologies that will benefit our great profession and the people and animals we serve.

Aaron J. Smiley, DVM
Veterinary Leadership Team
5030 South Scatterfield Road
Anderson, IN 46013, USA

E-mail address:
asmiley@vetcor.com

Vet Clin Small Anim 52 (2022) ix
https://doi.org/10.1016/j.cvsm.2022.07.001
0195-5616/22/© 2022 Published by Elsevier Inc.

What Is Telemedicine, Telehealth, and Teletriage

Mark Cushing, JD

KEYWORDS

- Telemedicine • Telehealth • Teletriage • Health heritage

KEY POINTS

- Human health care paved the way and serves as an all-purpose model for veterinary telemedicine.
- Remote care addresses the needs of animal owners who cannot access in-person care and/or prefer a virtual engagement for other reasons.

INTRODUCTION

Human health care has used telemedicine or virtual care for over 30 years. One-by-one, state medical practice acts and state medical boards paved the way for patients to gain access to remote care through digital tools. Appalachian Kentucky and rural Oklahoma paved the way, with telehealth serving people who could not access in-person medical care on a regular basis. All of the issues facing veterinary telemedicine were visited and resolved in human health care's adoption of telehealth over the past few decades.

Veterinary telemedicine officially launched in 2016 and remains at an early stage. Although veterinarians have "practiced" telemedicine since telephones became commonplace, the full-scale adoption of telehealth tools is a recent phenomenon and has met resistance as happened with human health care. Veterinary telemedicine or telehealth basically means that the client and patient are in a different location than the veterinary professional (DVM or Vet tech/nurse) and communicate with each other in real time via video links or messaging/emails. Veterinary practices handle this with staff or outsource to one of many telemedicine platform companies.

Once a veterinarian client–patient relationship (VCPR) is created, then practices are free to communicate with clients through any means they choose, including telemedicine. Although human medicine allows doctors to start relationships with clients through telemedicine, veterinary medicine struggles with the issue. The 2019, 2020, and 2021 witnessed the emergence of 20+ telehealth platform companies enabling veterinary practices to outsource telehealth services in a variety of methods. Some

13802 North Scottsdale Road, Suite 151 - 25, Scottsdale, AZ 85254-340, USA
E-mail address: mark@animalpolicygroup.com

Vet Clin Small Anim 52 (2022) 1069–1080
https://doi.org/10.1016/j.cvsm.2022.06.004
0195-5616/22/© 2022 Elsevier Inc. All rights reserved.

vetsmall.theclinics.com

veterinary telehealth companies rely principally on messaging, others on real-time video engagements. Some limit services to teletriage or advice, whereas others engage in full-scale telemedicine where permitted. Some offer white label platforms for practices, and others are technology providers linking the pet owner to a third-party licensed veterinarian.

DEFINITIONS

When used in these guidelines, these words and phrases shall be capitalized and are defined as follows:

- *Animal* means any member of the animal kingdom other than humans, whether living or dead.
- *Client* means a Person who has entered into an agreement with a Veterinarian for the purposes of obtaining veterinary medical services in-person or by any means of communication.
- *Consultation* means when a Veterinarian receives advice or assistance in-person, or by any method of communication, from another veterinarian or other Person whose expertise, in the opinion of the Veterinarian, would benefit a Patient. Under any circumstance, the responsibility for the welfare of the Patient remains with the Veterinarian receiving Consultation.
- *Informed Consent* means the Veterinarian has informed the Client or the Client's authorized representative, in a manner understood by the Client or representative, of the diagnostic and treatment options, risk assessment, and prognosis, and the Client has consented to the recommended treatment.
- *General Advice* means any advice provided by a Veterinarian or Veterinary Technician via any method of communication within or outside of an established VCPR that is given in general terms and is not specific to an individual Animal, group of Animals, diagnosis, or treatment.
- *Jurisdiction* means any commonwealth, state, or territory, including the District of Columbia, of the USA, or any province of Canada.
- *Patient* means any Animal or group of Animals receiving veterinary care from a Veterinarian or Veterinary Technician.
- *Person* means any individual, firm, partnership, association, joint venture, cooperative, corporation, governmental body, or any other group, legal entity, or combination acting in concert, and whether or not acting as a principal, trustee, fiduciary, receiver, or as any kind of legal or personal representative, or as the successor in interest, assignee, agent, factor, servant, employee, director, officer, or any other representative of such Person.
- *Telehealth* is the overarching term that encompasses all uses of technology geared to remotely deliver health information or education. Telehealth encompasses a broad variety of technologies and tactics to deliver virtual medical, health, and education services. Telehealth is not a specific service, but a collection of tools which allow Veterinarians to enhance care and education delivery. Telehealth encompasses both Telemedicine and General Advice.
- *Telemedicine* is the remote delivery of health care services, such as health assessments or consultations, over the telecommunications infrastructure. It allows Veterinarians to evaluate, diagnose, and treat patients without the need for an in-person visit.
- *Teletriage* means emergency Animal care, including Animal poison control services, for immediate, potentially life-threatening Animal health situations (eg,

poison exposure mitigation, Animal CPR instructions, other critical life-saving treatment or advice).

- *Veterinarian* means an individual who is duly licensed to practice Veterinary Medicine under the Jurisdiction's practice act. When not capitalized means an individual who is duly licensed to practice Veterinary Medicine in another Jurisdiction.
- *VCPR* exists when:
  1. Both the Veterinarian and Client agree for the Veterinarian to assume responsibility for making medical judgments regarding the health of the Animal(s);
  2. The Veterinarian has sufficient knowledge of the Animal(s) to initiate at least a general or preliminary diagnosis of the medical condition of the Animal(s);
  3. The practicing Veterinarian is readily available for follow-up in case of adverse reactions or failure of the regimen of therapy.
- *Veterinary Technician* means an individual who is duly licensed to practice Veterinary Technology under the Jurisdiction's practice act.

Telehealth incorporates the use of technology for delivering health information, guidance, care, or education. Telehealth embraces a variety of tools to deliver virtual medicine, advice, or services.

Telemedicine is the remote delivery of health care or medical services, such as health assessments, diagnoses, prescriptions, and treatment plans through a digital infrastructure. This enables a veterinarian to evaluate, diagnose, and treat patients through virtual tools regardless of how the VCPR is established. A veterinarian with a VCPR may practice telemedicine. *But* a VCPR must be in place for telemedicine to take place. A veterinarian without a VCPR may not practice telemedicine. Whether the VCPR may be created via digital means is discussed in depth later in this article.

Teletriage generally involves advice or guidance by a veterinary technician or veterinarian for a pet owner to assist a pet owner in determining whether a veterinary visit, emergency visit, or at-home procedures are warranted to address a concern or question the pet owner has regarding a pet. Teletriage is not limited to emergency circumstances and may be conducted by a veterinarian or veterinary technician. Teletriage is *not* the practice of medicine via digital means. Without a VCPR in place, the advice must be general and not cross the line into a diagnosis, prognosis, or treatment.

THE DEVELOPMENT OF VETERINARY TELEMEDICINE: 2016 TO 2021

In 2016, the North American Veterinary Community formed the Veterinary Innovation Council (VIC) with an impressive array of sponsors and animal health leaders. For the next 2 years, VIC developed veterinary telemedicine policies and promoted its adoption through outreach to a host of organizations and practitioners. The essence of VICs model policy is that a virtual VCPR may be created based on the judgment of the individual veterinarian as to whether she has adequate information to begin assisting the pet owner and animal.

Among the interested organizations in VICs initiative was the American Association of Veterinary State Boards (AAVSB), led by CEO Jim Penrod. AAVSB began considering veterinary telemedicine, and the VCPR at its September 2016 annual conference in Scottsdale, Arizona, with representatives of the AVMA and VIC invited to present their views. AAVSB devoted 2 years to evaluation of these issues and formally voted to adopt a model telemedicine policy at its 2018 annual conference in Washington, DC. Here is the *AAVSB Model Policy*:

GUIDELINES FOR THE APPROPRIATE USE OF TELEHEALTH TECHNOLOGIES IN VETERINARY MEDICAL PRACTICE

Licensure

A Veterinarian or Veterinary Technician must be licensed by, or under the authority of, the Board of Veterinary Medicine in the Jurisdiction where the VCPR is established (location of Patient at time of VCPR establishment).

Any veterinarian who is licensed in another Jurisdiction, or any Person whose expertise, in the opinion of the Veterinarian with an established VCPR, would benefit an Animal, and who is consulting with the Veterinarian, is exempt from licensure in this Jurisdiction, provided such service is limited to such Consultation.

Evaluation and Treatment of the Patient(s)

The Veterinarian must use sound professional judgment to determine whether using Telehealth is suitable each time veterinary services are provided and only furnish medical advice or treatment via Telemedicine when it is medically appropriate. A Veterinarian using Telemedicine must take appropriate steps to establish the VCPR, obtain Informed Consent from the Client, and conduct all necessary Patient evaluations consistent with currently acceptable standards of care. Some Patient presentations are appropriate for the utilization of Telemedicine as a component of, or in lieu of, hands-on medical care, whereas others are not.

The Veterinarian must take appropriate precautions to safeguard the confidentiality of a Client's or Patient's records. Such includes ensuring that technology and physical settings used as part of Telemedicine services are compliant with Jurisdictional or federal requirements.

The Veterinarian must ensure that the Client is aware of the Veterinarian's identity, location, and Jurisdiction's license number and licensure status. Evidence documenting Informed Consent for the use of Telemedicine must be obtained and maintained in the medical record.

Continuity of Care/Medical Records

Veterinarians must maintain appropriate medical records that contain sufficient information for continued care and are compliant with Jurisdictional requirements. Documentation of the telemedicine encounter should be readily available on request by the Client.

Emergency Services

Teletriage may be performed by a Veterinarian or Veterinary Technician without establishing a VCPR or obtaining Informed Consent to provide emergency, potentially life-saving Telemedicine services.

Prescribing Medications

Prescribing medications in-person or via Telemedicine requires a VCPR and is at the professional discretion of the Veterinarian. The indication, appropriateness, and safety considerations for each prescription issued in association with Telemedicine services must be evaluated by the Veterinarian in accordance with all Jurisdictional and federal laws and standards of care.

Telemedicine Service Requirements

A provider of Telemedicine services must ensure that the Client is aware of the Veterinarian's identity, location, and Jurisdiction's license number and licensure status and should provide to Clients a clear mechanism to:

1. Access, supplement, and amend Client-provided contact information and health information about the Patient.
2. Register complaints with the appropriate Board of Veterinary Medicine or other regulatory body.

The *AVMAs model policy* insists that the VCPR may only be established via an in-person examination of the animal as follows:

"Telehealth is the overarching term that encompasses all uses of technology geared to remotely deliver health information or education. Telemedicine is the use of medical information exchanged from one site to another via electronic communications regarding a patient's clinical health status.

Telemedicine is a tool that may be used to augment the practice of veterinary medicine. The AVMA is committed to ensuring access to the convenience and benefits afforded by telemedicine while promoting the responsible provision of high-quality veterinary medical care. Veterinary care, whether delivered through electronic or other means, should be provided with professionalism.

The AVMA encourages the development of smart-device applications, other platforms, and technologies that appropriately help connect current or lapsed clients and patients with veterinarians. In addition, veterinarians may use emerging technologies to enhance their accessibility and client communications and support exceptional patient care.

Given the current state of technological capabilities, available research, and the current state and federal regulatory landscape, the AVMA believes that veterinary telemedicine should only be conducted within an existing VCPR, with the exception for advice given in an emergency until that patient can be seen by a veterinarian.

Most states and the AVMAs Principles of Veterinary Medical Ethics require a VCPR for a veterinarian to diagnose, prescribe medication, or otherwise treat an animal. Federal law also requires a VCPR for prescribing extra-label drugs for animals and issuing Veterinary Feed Directives.

Under the VCPR, a veterinarian assumes responsibility for making medical judgments and ensures that he or she has sufficient knowledge of the patient to initiate at least a general or preliminary diagnosis of the medical condition of the patient.

The VCPR ensures that a veterinarian is readily available for follow-up evaluation or has arranged for veterinary emergency coverage and continuing care and treatment. The veterinarian is expected to provide oversight of treatment, compliance, and outcome, as well as document the patient's continuing care and treatment in the medical record. The animal owner's consent for the use of telemedicine must also be obtained and documented. Without a VCPR, any advice provided through electronic means should be general and not specific to a patient, diagnosis, or treatment.

The AVMA recognizes that future policy in this area will be informed by evidence-based research on the impact of telemedicine on access to care and patient safety. With the exception of emergency teletriage, including poison control services, the AVMA opposes remote consulting, including telemedicine, offered directly to the public when the intent is to diagnose and/or treat a patient in the absence of a VCPR.

A veterinarian with a VCPR has the professional discretion to consult with specialists or other consultants. The specialist or consultant should not be required to hold an active veterinary medical license in the state within which the veterinarian with the VCPR practices or within which the patient or client resides." Canada's Ontario province in June of 2018 adopted the first full-scale telemedicine policy in a practice act and allowed the formation of a virtual VCPR. Ontario's Veterinary Medical Association worked with the governing board to develop this policy and educate veterinarians about *what* they could do and *how* to do it. The Ontario VMA also followed up with surveys of practitioners to assess usage, reactions, and impact on practices. These surveys generally were very positive and to date no pet owner in Ontario has reported any harm to a pet through the usage of telemedicine. Telemedicine advocates in the United States often cite 15-million person Ontario as the best laboratory demonstrating the efficacy and safety of telemedicine.

Overview of the Veterinarian-Client-Patient Relationship and Its History

Creation of the VCPR throughout the United States was not driven by state legislators independently, but rather at the behest of organized veterinary medicine. As you may expect, the precise conditions for creating a working relationship between pet owners or food animal producers and veterinarians were not topics of keen interest, and ranchers, farmers, and pet owners were not rubbing their hands anxiously trying to determine if they had a state-approved "official" relationship with their veterinarian. However, when states developed veterinary practice acts, all but a few jurisdictions decided to establish some framework for determining what a licensed veterinarian can and cannot do. And this foundation included a definition of when and how a veterinarian "legally" becomes the veterinarian for a particular animal, namely through VCPR. The purpose of a VCPR was to provide a legal basis for a state veterinary medical board to take action against a veterinarian if an animal was harmed due to negligence or violation of a veterinary law or regulation.

Veterinarians are not required to report to their state veterinary medical board when they have established a VCPR with a particular animal owner, and state veterinary medical boards do not have investigators whose job it is to monitor whether veterinarians properly initiate a VCPR. For decades, the topic of a VCPR rarely was mentioned in state veterinary medical boards or state and national VMA meetings. Frankly, the VCPR was something of an academic topic, although it was a baseline determination in state board actions against a veterinarian. Interestingly, there is no evidence that the few states without a VCPR have lower standards of care or greater incidence of veterinarian misconduct or malpractice.

The VCPR became prominent in veterinary medicine with the arrival of telemedicine in 2016. Human health care faced the same issue: could a doctor–client relationship be established virtually or only through in-person examinations? All 50 states now allow a virtual doctor–client relationship, and now veterinary medicine faces the same choice. Most states insist on an in-person examination, with only Idaho, Michigan, New Jersey, Oklahoma, and Virginia allowing a virtual VCPR and New York not requiring any form of VCPR. A host of economic and political issues swirl around this topic, but the medical question is whether a veterinarian should be allowed to trust his or her judgment that a digital engagement with the pet owner and animal provides enough information to get started in caring for the patient.

How Does Each State Handle the Telemedicine Veterinarian-Client-Patient Relationship?

There are six categories for how states handle the VCPR, either through practice acts or board regulations. Let us examine each one.

1. *No VCPR provisions whatsoever.* In these states, the veterinary practice act makes no reference to or use the term VCPR. In other words, there are no legal criteria for formation of a VCPR (Michigan and New York).
2. *Virtual VCPR is allowed.* These states expressly permit the formation of a virtual VCPR, often with conditions: MI, OK, ID, VA, NJ, and FL. Michigan does this

through veterinary board regulations, and the others through the practice act. Florida expressly bans prescriptions of medications if the VCPR is only virtual. Michigan's regulations provide an example of guardrails or conditions that must be honored in order to establish a virtual VCPR as follows.

R 338.4901a Telehealth services

Rule 1a. (1) A veterinarian providing a telehealth service shall do all of the following:

   a. Ensure that the client knows the identity and contact information of the veterinarian providing the telehealth service. Upon request, the veterinarian shall provide his or her licensure information including the name of the state where he or she is licensed and his or her license number.

   b. Ensure that the technology method and equipment used to provide telehealth services complies with all current privacy-protection laws.

   c. Employ sound professional judgment to determine whether using telehealth is an appropriate method for delivering medical advice or treatment to the animal patient.

   d. Have sufficient knowledge of the animal patient to render telehealth services demonstrated by satisfying one of the following:

      i. Have recently examined the animal patient in person or have obtained current knowledge of the animal patient through the use of instrumentation and diagnostic equipment through which images and medical records may be transmitted electronically.

3. *Absolutely no telemedicine VCPR*. The veterinary practice act unequivocally bans a VCPR through telemedicine: CA, CT, GA, IL, MS, NV, NC, TN, TX, UT, and WA. Here is sample language from Texas:

   Sec. 801.351. EXISTENCE OF VETERINARIAN-CLIENT-PATIENT RELATIONSHIP.

   c. A veterinarian–client–patient relationship may not be established solely by telephone or electronic means.

4. In order for a veterinarian to create a VCPR with an animal, the client and the patient must have been "seen" or the veterinarian must have become "acquainted with" the animal: AZ, CO, IN, LA, ME, RI, and SD. The definition of "seen" or "become acquainted with" has never been tested with a veterinary medical board or court. Some telemedicine advocates are eager to explore whether the animal could be seen or acquainted with through real-time video technologies.

5. *The veterinarian must have examined or physically examined the animal before a VCPR can be established*: AL, AR, CT, DC, HI, KS, KY, MD, MN, MO, MT, NE, NH, NM, ND, OH, OR, PA, SC, VT, WV, WI, and WY. "Examined" or "physically examined" has always been construed to mean an in-person or clinic visit.

6. *Time limits on When Animal Last Seen* (VCPR lasts for 1 year after animal is physically seen): FL, GA, ID, OR, SC, TN, WA, and CA (for purposes of a prescription). This prescriptive approach requires a pet owner to bring a pet annually to the clinic. Here is sample language from South Carolina:

   120-1. Definitions.

   "Veterinarian–client–patient relationship" means:

   (6) The veterinarian–client–patient relationship lapses when the licensee has not seen the animal within 1 year.

DVM LIABILITY AND OTHER ETHICAL AND PRACTICE CONSIDERATIONS

Veterinarians are bound by the same standard of care whether their services are delivered in-person or via telemedicine. This is a hard and fast rule, which means that telemedicine cannot be used as a vehicle for substandard care. This is a crucial element in a veterinarian's judgment that he or she has enough information through a digital encounter to begin caring for a patient. If a key piece of information or viewing cannot be accomplished through a virtual encounter, then best practices call for an in-person visit.

The VVCA has developed a practical set of tools or guidelines for veterinarians to deploy in a virtual engagement. These are presented below as the best example of rules of the road for telemedicine practitioners, including an Informed Consent form.

BEST PRACTICES: LEGAL AND ETHICAL ISSUES WITH DELIVERING VIRTUAL CARE

There is a need for clarity on the following issues by State Boards in regard to best practices Legal and Ethical Issues with Delivering Virtual care. Check with your state, territory, or country to learn the rules and regulations that apply in your area, especially pertaining to your:

a. Veterinary practice act.
b. Pharmacy act.
c. Licensure and credentialing.
d. Record retention.
e. Client confidentiality.
f. Federal laws and regulations, including FDA, USDA, DEA, OSHA, and so forth.

All telemedicine must adhere to the respective rules and regulations of the given state, territory, or country. Defining the VCPR such that it is precise enough to provide consistent and predictable guidance to the licensees. If a physical examination is required:

a. Is it "personally acquainted" examination or can it be done by another vet in the practice or licensed professional such as nurse or technician?
b. Is it a "physical" examination or can it be a "virtual" examination?
c. How long ago does the PE have to have been done so that it is still valid to maintain the VCPR?
d. Does the PE have to be related to the condition for which the telemedicine consult is being requested?

Development of Virtual Care Standards of Care by State Boards and Experts Within the Veterinary Community

a. Clarity for the State Board as to what differentiates "teleadvice/teletriage" from telemedicine

Staff Utilizing Virtual Care Should Be Trained to Do So Properly

a. Ensure every shift has capacity for those assigned to be fully dedicated to telemedicine if needed.

Identify and frame opportunities for appropriate use of telemedicine, including

a. Preventative care
b. Hospice and end-of-life care
c. Client education
d. Teletriage
e. For clients/patients located in underserved areas
f. To assist in monitoring patients in isolation

g. Recommending patients that are not suitable patients for telemedicine to be seen in-person.

Licensing Issues

a. Determine how VCPR is established
b. Determine where veterinarian has to be licensed
c. Determine continuing education requirements specific to telemedicine if practice includes telemedicine consultation
d. Determine whether any veterinarian who is licensed in another Jurisdiction, or any Person whose expertise, in the opinion of the Veterinarian with an established VCPR, would benefit an Animal, and who is consulting with the Veterinarian, is exempt from licensure in this Jurisdiction.

Medical Record Keeping

I. Integration with platforms of service providers assisting with data collection and monetization of telemedicine consultations
  A. Confidentiality: released as required or allowed by law or by consent of the owner of the patient.
  B. Data security: encryption of data during transmission and at rest.
  C. Data integration and retrievability.
  D. Data need to be maintained and available in accordance with state laws and regulations.
II. Copies of all patient-related electronic communications
  A. Client–veterinarian communication
  B. Prescriptions
  C. Test results
  D. Evaluations
  E. Consultations
  F. Records of past care
III. Instructions obtained or produced in connection with the
  A. utilization of telemedicine services
IV. Signed Informed Consent form
V. Monetize telemedicine services appropriately
  A. Expressing professional expertise
  B. Client convenience
  C. Animal health and welfare
  D. Secure collection of payment for services

Practices and virtual care service providers should develop, maintain, and implement written policies and procedures for documentation, maintenance, and transmission of the records of encounters using telemedicine services. Such policies and procedures should address:

1. Veterinarians and virtual care service providers should provide current pet owners with a copy of the patient's records on request in a timely manner.
2. Privacy.
3. Personnel who will process messages.
4. Hours of operation.
5. Types of transactions that will be permitted electronically.
6. Required patient information to be included in the communication, such as name, species, breed, sex, weight, and presenting complaint.
7. Archival and retrieval.

8. Quality oversight mechanisms.

Policies and procedures for veterinary medical record privacy, data management, and security should be:

1. Written.
2. Periodically reviewed and, as needed, updated.
3. Maintained in an accessible and readily available manner.
4. Veterinarians should be aware that they can use their own data for research, education, marketing, public good, and so forth, when the data are anonymized.
5. Veterinarians using third party vendors should be aware of how those vendors are using data obtained from their clients.

Malpractice Insurance

a. Ensure telemedicine services provided by the insured are covered
b. Assess the risks of using virtual care platform vendors, such as:
    i. How do they maintain medical record confidentiality?
    ii. How do they capture and store information, and for how long?
    iii. Do they have insurance, and does the insurance protect the health care provider?
    iv. Does the health care provider's primary malpractice insurance protect against vendor negligence?
c. Be aware that malpractice insurance may not cover practitioners treating patients in states in which they are not licensed.
    i. Practitioners should be aware of how each state regulates VCPR and telemedicine services.
d. Check with your professional liability carrier for any additional recommendations it may have pertaining to providing telemedicine services.

Client Communication Tailored to the Provision of Telemedicine

a. Be sure to reply to owners in a timely, professional manner.
b. If your practice does not have the capacity to dedicate someone to telemedicine, establish specific time(s) during the workday to incorporate telemedicine consultations.

Client Consent Forms Should Address the Following Main Concepts

a. Identification of the client, the patient, the practitioner, and the practitioner's credentials, location, and Jurisdiction's license number and licensure status.
b. Introduction to telemedicine.
c. Record keeping.
d. Hold harmless clause for information lost because of technical failures.
e. Requirement for express client consent to forward medical records to a third party if needed.
f. The client understands the potential risks and benefits of telemedicine.
g. The client understands that the laws that protect privacy and the confidentiality of traditional medical information also apply to telemedicine.
h. The client understands that no information obtained in the use of telemedicine which identifies the client or patient will be disclosed to researchers or other entities without the client's consent.
i. The client understands that they have the right to withhold or withdraw their consent to the use of telemedicine in the course of patient care at any time.

j. The client engaging in telemedicine understands that in-person options are available for treatment and care.
k. The client understands that there will be a plan for ongoing care.
l. The client understands that there will be a plan for alternative care in the case of an emergency or technological malfunction.
m. The client understands that it is the role of the veterinarian to determine whether the presenting complaint is appropriate for a telemedicine encounter.
n. The client has the ability to register complaints with the appropriate Board of Veterinary Medicine or other regulatory body.

Requirements for Prescribing Through Telemedicine

a. Determine if the state in which you are providing services requires an in-person physical examination to prescribe medication through telemedicine.
b. The indication, appropriateness, and safety considerations for each prescription issued in association with telemedicine services must be evaluated by the veterinarian in accordance with all jurisdictional and federal laws and standards of care.

Client Consent Form for Telemedicine Services

Telemedicine involves the use of electronic communications to enable animal health care providers at different locations to share individual patient medical information for the purpose of improving animal care. Providers may include primary care veterinarians, specialists, and/or subspecialists. The information may be used for diagnosis, therapy, follow-up, and/or education and may include any of the following:

1. Patient medical records
2. Medical images
3. Real-time text communication
4. Live two-way audio and video
5. Output data from medical devices and sound and video files

Electronic systems used will incorporate network and software security protocols to protect the confidentiality of client and patient's identification and imaging data and will include measures to safeguard the data and to ensure its integrity against intentional or unintentional corruption.

Expected Benefits

1. Improved access to medical care by enabling a client and patient to remain at a remote site, whereas the veterinarian obtains test results and consults from other veterinarians at distant/other sites.
2. More efficient medical evaluation and management.
3. Obtaining expertise of a distant specialist.

Possible Risks

As with any medical procedure, there are potential risks associated with the use of telemedicine. These risks include, but may not be limited to:

1. In rare cases, information transmitted may not be sufficient (eg, poor resolution of images) to allow for appropriate medical decision-making by the veterinarian and consultant(s);
2. Delays in medical evaluation and treatment could occur due to deficiencies or failures of the equipment;
3. In rare instances, security protocols could fail, causing a breach of privacy of personal medical information;

4. In rare cases, a lack of access to complete medical records may result in adverse drug interactions or allergic reactions or other judgment errors;

Pros and Cons and a Look to the Future

1. *Concern*: Clients will not convert from free telemedicine to paid telemedicine. Many veterinarians confess that they have provided free advice over the phone to clients for years. This is a common practice and often important to maintain a client's loyalty. However, many health professionals and others charge fees for telephone consults, and pet owners have shown that they will pay for valuable advice to help them manage their pet's health care. Experience proves this barrier may be overcome quickly.
2. *Concern*: Technology is too difficult to quickly use. This makes the case for using one of the 20+ telemedicine platform companies that take care of the technology piece for you. If you do not have staff trained or interested in managing the delivery of telemedicine or telehealth services, outsource it.
3. *Concern*: Veterinarians do not have time to see remote cases because the in-clinic calendar is full. This is the most powerful rationale for outsourcing, particularly with the large number of licensed veterinarians working from home, often part-time.
4. *Concern*: Clients do not want telemedicine. Every survey or study proves the opposite. Millennials and Generation Zs own the greatest number of pets, and they manage every part of their life through digital tools. Smartphones rule the world. Most of the time they want advice or questions answered about pet behavior or conditions, and avoiding an unnecessary trip to the clinic is welcome news.
5. *Concern*: Offering telemedicine will increase my professional liability. Standards of care are the same and just check with your liability carrier about coverage for telemedicine services.
6. *Concern*: Telemedicine decrease medical standards. We covered this earlier. The standards are the same for in-person and telemedicine care.
7. *Concern*: My license might be in jeopardy. Follow your veterinary practice act and veterinary medical board regulations and you will be safe. Telehealth and teletriage are legal everywhere. Once a VCPR is in place you may practice telemedicine with any client.

SUMMARY

Telemedicine is a tool alongside other tools veterinarians possess to address client needs and deliver quality medicine. For pet owners who cannot access a clinic, telemedicine is the only option or their pet goes without health care.

DISCLOSURE

Provide services to over 30 clients in animal health, animal welfare and veterinary education sectors. In addition, service over 30 animal health companies, organizations, animal welfare organizations and veterinary colleges related to accreditation.

Teletriage-How Remote Advice Provides Better Care

Katherine Donahue, DVM

KEYWORDS

- Teletriage • Advice • Remote • Veterinary

KEY POINTS

- Teletriage improves access to care.
  - Animal owners in underserved areas can engage with veterinary professionals.
  - Animal owners can start therapy in emergency situations while on their way to in-person care.
- Teletriage provides a financial benefit to veterinary practices.
  - Nonemergent problems can be scheduled appropriately, leaving additional time open for urgent or emergency cases to be seen.
  - Teletriage improves customer satisfaction which leads to improved customer loyalty.
- Teletriage reduces the burden at emergency practices.
  - Nonemergent concerns can be diverted back to the general practitioner.
  - Resources can be directed toward emergent cases when there are fewer nonemergent concerns to deal with.

DEFINITIONS

Teleadvice: the provision of any health information, opinion, guidance, or recommendation concerning prudent future actions that are not specific to a particular patient's health, illness, or injury. This is general advice that is not intended to diagnose, prognose, treat, correct, change, alleviate, or prevent animal disease, illness, pain, deformity, defect, injury, or other physical, dental, or mental conditions.[1]

Teletriage: the safe, appropriate, and timely assessment and management (immediate referral to a veterinarian or not) of animal patients via electronic consultation with their owners. In assessing patient condition electronically, the assessor determines urgency and the need for immediate referral to a veterinarian, based on the owner's (or responsible party's) report of history and clinical signs, sometimes supplemented by visual (e.g., photographs, video) information. A diagnosis is not rendered. The essence of teletriage is to make good and safe decisions regarding a patient's disposition (immediate referral to a veterinarian or not) under conditions of uncertainty and urgency.[1]

GuardianVets, 1801 West Belle Plaine Suite 205, Chicago, IL 60613, USA
E-mail address: katherine@guardianvets.com

Vet Clin Small Anim 52 (2022) 1081–1086
https://doi.org/10.1016/j.cvsm.2022.06.001
0195-5616/22/© 2022 Elsevier Inc. All rights reserved.
vetsmall.theclinics.com

Veterinary professional: A person with veterinary medical training who is not a veterinarian.

COMPARING HUMAN AND VETERINARY TRIAGE

Human medical triage began as an approach to maximizing human survival in mass casualty events, most commonly seen on the battlefield. Injured soldiers would be sorted according to the severity of their wounds, and the ones who were expected to survive would be prioritized ahead of those with mortal wounds. Soldiers with minor injuries were treated last.

Triage in veterinary medicine is very similar and is most commonly utilized at emergency clinics. Veterinary teletriage employs the same general process with 2 variations. First, a single animal is typically evaluated. Secondly, the veterinary professional is not in the same physical location as the animal and its owner.

VETERINARY TELETRIAGE TECHNOLOGY

Any secure communication device can be used for teletriage as long as the animal owner can relay enough pertinent data to the veterinarian professional to make a proper judgment about the urgency of care. For years teletriage was confined to the telephone and was reliant on a client's verbal description of the animal's problem. Today, technology allows the veterinary profession to get first-hand information through high definition videos and photos. This has dramatically improved the quality of teletriage.

For example, a dog owner is concerned about her Great Dane's sudden onset of lameness. She engages a veterinary professional via teletriage to seek advice as to whether she should take her dog to the emergency clinic immediately or if she can wait for an appointment with her regular veterinarian. Teletriage confined to a phone call is dependent on the animal owner's description of the limp. The owner might describe a mild limp as severe resulting in an unnecessary trip to the emergency room. If, on the other hand, the owner sends a video of the limp, the veterinary professional can assess the severity of the limp first hand, and make a better recommendation. As technology evolves, veterinary professionals will be able to obtain more first-hand data and the quality of teletriage will continue to improve.

WHO CAN PROVIDE VETERINARY TELETRIAGE?

Veterinary teletriage is not the practice of medicine and the laws regulating who can provide it are sparse. At a minimum, the person providing triage ought to have easy access to a licensed veterinarian to ensure the animal owner receives medically appropriate information. Formal teletriage training decreases the risk that a veterinary professional will inadvertently move from teletriage to telemedicine. This is important because the evolution of a conversation from teletriage to telemedicine has legal ramifications.

The "rule of thumb" when offering teletriage is to not diagnose, prognose, or prescribe. These 3 actions are the most common boundaries that differentiate teletriage from telemedicine. Most recognize that a veterinarian has the sole authority to diagnose, but sometimes veterinary professionals do not realize when they inadvertently diagnose a patient.

For example, an email is sent from an animal owner that contains a video of her dog making intermittent, abnormal, and respiratory noises. The client wants to know if she needs to have her dog seen by the veterinarian as soon as possible, or if it is something she can monitor until she finds a convenient time to schedule an exam. It is acceptable for the veterinary professional to let the owner know that the dog does not need to be seen immediately, but the veterinary professional cannot tell the owner that the sound in the video is a reverse sneeze. Understanding the nuance of what constitutes a diagnosis is critical to maintaining compliance with regulations.

A prognosis is the likely course of a disease, and it is a commonly overlooked restriction of teletriage. In most states, a prognosis is considered part of the practice of veterinary medicine, but veterinary professionals can unknowingly offer animal owners a prognosis for the patient. As an example, an animal owner who has a cat that is urinating outside the litter pan contacts the veterinary professional via teletriage to learn and get advice about what can be conducted in the environment to ameliorate the problem. The professional can gather information and discuss common causes of inappropriate urination, but she cannot speculate about the likelihood that the cat will start using the litter pan again. The veterinary professional cannot inform the owner that her cat is going to be fine, or on the other hand, that the cat will never use the litter pan again, resulting in a shortened life span. Both statements constitute a prognosis and are outside the scope of teletriage.

Finally, prescribing medications is the most intuitive restriction of teletriage. The veterinary professional cannot refill or offer an animal owner a new prescription. This restriction is sometimes inadvertently overlooked by veterinary professionals in regards to chronic medication or preventative medication, but a veterinarian must be involved in the decision to prescribe. Teletriage is often provided outside of veterinary medicine by people at grooming salons, pet food stores, boarding kennels, and training facilities. This can be good and bad. On the positive side, a groomer who talks to her client over the phone about the cat's debris filled ears can direct the animal owner to seek veterinary care. On the negative side, a pet store employee might recommend a new type of dog food over the phone for a dog who is a "finicky eater" without considering that the dog needs to be evaluated by the veterinarian because it is overweight and ought to consume fewer calories.

Veterinary emergency room experience or extensive general practice experience best prepares a veterinary professional for teletriage. During the teletriage process, triage providers must make quick decisions about the immediate need for care during an emergency situation. In person emergency experience helps the veterinary professional "keep her cool" when she is dealing with a stressful remote situation.

Veterinary teletriage can be provided by a third-party. An offsite teletriage team will reduce the staffing burden for the local clinic and free up time to offer more in person care. Utilizing a third-party provider has the additional benefit of allowing veterinary teams to rest when the clinic is closed, as opposed to providing the triage themselves. It is important to know the third party provider's protocols and how information will be exchanged between the remote and local teams. Additionally, consider the training, experience, and licensure of the veterinary professionals that are employed by a third party triage service.

Artificial intelligence is starting to emerge as another teletriage tool. Algorithms are being built that can gather data and move through sophisticated decision trees to help animal owners make better medical decisions for their animals. Technology will never replace the veterinary professional, but it has the potential to increase teletriage efficiency and reduce mistakes.

THE VETERINARY TELETRIAGE WORKFLOW

The teletriage process is almost always initiated by the animal owner and typically follows the following workflow.

1. Gather animal owner information
2. Gather animal information
3. Determine stability of animal
4. Determine urgency of care
5. Schedule exam with veterinarian

   The most important aspect of the veterinary teletriage process is to quickly and concisely gather relevant information. This includes a caller's name, phone number, animal information,and the chief complaint that motivated the animal owner to reach out. Documentation is critical because teletriage cases almost always get passed to another veterinary professional or to a veterinarian. A lack of documentation or poor documentation will increase the risk of medical errors and/or frustrate the animal owner if she has to repeat information to each new veterinary professional involved in the case.

TELETRIAGE REDUCES THE COST OF VETERINARY MEDICAL CARE

According to data from 2018, the average cost of an emergency room visit for a pet can range between $800-$1500.[2] Teletriage can reduce the cost of animal ownership by keeping non-emergent cases out of the emergency room. For example, an animal owner who does not have access to teletriage is concerned that her young dog with diarrhea needs to be seen by a veterinarian immediately. She is worried that the dog will become dehydrated before she can get in to see her regular veterinarian. The ER veterinarian evaluates the puppy and is confident the patient is in good health and will recover quickly. The owner leaves the ER with peace of mind and the burden of the cost of emergency care. If the same owner would have had access to teletriage, she could have received the same peace of mind at a fraction of the cost, and the ER could have used its resources for the truly emergent cases.

TELETRIAGE IN EMERGENCY CLINICS

Teletriage in emergency clinics is an important part of providing emergency services and managing workflows. When teletriage is provided to incoming callers, patient loads can be managed more efficiently. Callers with less critical animals can be prepared for longer wait times. This results in less frustrated animal owners.

   Teletriage also helps with emergency room resource allocation. Often, veterinary emergency rooms are at capacity for cage space, surgical services, or veterinary team members. If an animal owner can receive triage over the phone prior to arriving at the ER, he can be diverted to another facility that can offer faster care.

MANAGING THE ANIMAL OWNER DURING TELETRIAGE

Animal owners in need of urgent care for their pet are often upset, abrupt, hysterical, or rude. Veterinary professionals providing teletriage need to be prepared to assist owners quickly, consistently, and meet frantic or emotional language with calm, directed questions and concise instructions.

TELETRIAGE KEEPS NON-EMERGENT CASES AT HOME PRACTICE

Providing after-hours triage services for clients strengthens the bond clients feel with both their veterinarian and their home practice. Clients appreciate the practice support provided to them when the practice is closed. Clients are not left on their own to figure out if their pet is experiencing a true emergency. They engage with an expert who helps them make the next right medical decision for their animal.

TELETRIAGE CAN PROVIDE LIFESAVING ADVICE ON THE WAY TO IN-PERSON EMERGENCY CARE

Teletriage and teleadvice can be lifesaving in multiple types of veterinary emergencies. Choking, severe hemorrhage, and cardiopulmonary resuscitation are examples of emergent presentations that can be positively impacted by a trained veterinary professional relaying lifesaving instructions to an owner, caregiver, or bystander.

A dog can obstruct its airway with common household items such as rubber balls, bones, or corn cobs. The eXternal eXtraction Technique (XXT)[3] is a technique for relieving complete airway obstructions in an unconscious dog that can be performed by an owner with the instruction of a veterinary professional. This technique involves positioning a dog on its back and stroking the throat in a J-shaped movement to push the foreign object antegrade.

Severe hemorrhage is another emergency that a veterinary professional via teletriage can have a profound impact on the outcome of the case. Some owners panic at the sight of even a small amount of blood and become helpless toward their animal in need. But if that same owner has access to teletriage she can be instructed on how to best manage the hemorrhage and where the closest ER clinic is so that her animal has a better chance of survival.

CPR (cardiopulmonary resuscitation) is an additional life saving measure that owners or caregivers can potentially provide to their pet when there is cardiac or respiratory arrest. Unfortunately, very few people are trained in pet CPR.[4] A calm voice on the other end of the phone relaying CPR instructions to an owner can change the outcome of the cardiac or respiratory arrest case. Even if the pet does die, owners who have been empowered to intervene appropriately are spared the feelings of utter helplessness that can intensify the grief of losing a pet.

TELETRIAGE CAN PROVIDE ACCESS TO CARE FOR REMOTE LOCATIONS

Animal owners who live in remote geographic areas often have considerably fewer options for veterinary care compared to those who live in more populated areas. The Toronto Humane Society reported that approximately 40% of pets in Canada do not currently have an established relationship with a veterinarian, and that many owners live over a 100 kilometers or more away from the nearest veterinary clinic.[5] Teletriage provides the animal owner with a veterinary professional that can help owners assess the timelines around the need for care when physically going to a veterinary clinic is not a feasible option. Lifesaving instructions can be provided while owners are in the process of seeking care.

SUMMARY

In summation, teletriage and remote advice provide better care for our animal patients and animal owners. This is accomplished in multiple ways. First, teletriage helps keep non-emergent cases out of the emergency room and reduces the burden on our emergency care providers. Second, it solidifies the bond that clients have with their home practice. Supporting clients during legitimate or perceived after-hours emergencies improves customer loyalty. Third, veterinary teletriage can provide lifesaving advice on the way to in person emergency care. This can be the difference between life and death for certain cases.

Finally, teletriage services improve access to care for all, but particularly for those in remote areas. Many areas of the country face shortages in veterinary services. Assistance from a veterinary professional in determining the urgency and acuity of a clinical presentation can be critical. Teletriage is a powerful tool that can improve the delivery of veterinary care and support the professionals who protect animal health and relieve animal suffering.

CLINICS CARE POINTS

- Veterinary teletriage is best performed by licensed veterinary professionals, such as veterinarians and veterinary nurses.
- Those individuals that provide veterinary teletriage should take care not to inadvertently practice veterinary medicine by providing a diagnosis or prognosis.
- There are certain caller concerns that always warrant an immediate, in-person exam by a veterinarian and those include but are not limited to; active on-going seizures, collapse, dyspnea, and major trauma.

DISCLOSURE

Dr K. Donahue is the Veterinary Medical Director at GuardianVets, a leading veterinary teletriage provider.

REFERENCES

1. AVMA. Available at: https://www.avma.org/resources-tools/practice-management/telehealth-telemedicine-veterinary-practice/veterinary-telehealth-basics.
2. Are you prepared for a pet emergency? Most Americans are not," Carmen Reinicke, 6/14/18. Available at: https://www.cnbc.com/2018/06/14/are-you-prepared-for-a-pet-emergency-most-americans-are-not.html.
3. Robin Van Metre VMD, Dennis T, Tim C Jr. DVM, Diplomate ACVS Emeritus, Charter Diplomate ACVECC, FCCM; KaLee Pasek, DVM; Jo-Anne Brenner, EMT-Tactical, NREMT-I, K9™ Medic Executive Director and Founder. Intervention for Choking in an Unconscious Dog: XXT – eXternal eXtraction Technique. 2018. Available at: https://veterinarypartner.vin.com/default.aspx?pid=19239&id=8871225.
4. Craig B, North Kentucky Tribune. Do you know pet first aid? Survey finds just two percent are prepared for a pet's illness or injury. 2021. Available at:https://www.nkytribune.com/2021/05/do-you-know-pet-first-aid-survey-finds-just-two-percent-are-prepared-for-a-pets-illness-or-injury/. .
5. Toronto Humane Society. Access To Care. Available at: https://www.torontohumanesociety.com/purpose/ensuring-access-to-care/.

Wearable Devices in Veterinary Health Care

Ashley Mitek, DVM, MS, DACVAA[a],*, Dylan Jones, MS[b,c,d], Andrew Newell, BSBA[d,e], Samantha Vitale, DVM, MS, DACVIM (Neurology)[f]

KEYWORDS

- Wearables • IoT • IoVT • Telehealth • Virtual veterinary care • Telemedicine
- Teleconsulting • AI

KEY POINTS

- Wearable devices will increasingly play an important role in veterinary health care.
- Veterinarians should have a working knowledge of how these devices may help them practice the best veterinary care possible.
- Overcoming adoption barriers is a current challenge but market share will continue to increase as pet owners and veterinarians recognize the value of wearables.
- Wearables can assist with the remote diagnosis of common diseases and assist in triage scenarios.
- Early recognition of disease is an area where wearables show great promise.

INTRODUCTION

The wearable revolution is coming to a veterinary practice near you. If you have not worked with a client yet who wants to use a wearable on their pet, you will soon. Wearables have been affecting human health care for decades and have mostly entered the veterinary health-care market through consumers/pet owners. Wearable sensors became more prevalent in industrialized societies in the 2010s and initially had a fitness focus.[1] These pet owners are the "early adopters" in a bell-curve distribution of people adopting new technology. Moving toward the center of the curve, where we see mass adoption, will require more integration of the technology into veterinary medicine. Wearable devices are expected to play a major role in the remote and continuous monitoring of health and the early detection of disease.[2] Adoption of this technology often shifts health-care ecosystems toward a patient-centered, transparent, and proactive culture.

[a] Co-Founder, Stratocyte.com, Owner, AnesthesiaDiva.com; [b] Texas Christian University; [c] United States Air Force, Veteran; [d] Animal Cloud Device Connectivity, Inc; [e] University of Colorado, Boulder; [f] Stratocyte.com
* Corresponding author. 48-113 Angel Wing Peak, Glacier National Park, MT, USA.
E-mail address: diva@anesthesiadiva.com

Vet Clin Small Anim 52 (2022) 1087–1098
https://doi.org/10.1016/j.cvsm.2022.05.001
0195-5616/22/© 2022 Elsevier Inc. All rights reserved.

This article reviews the use of wearable technology for veterinary patients, and the future of wearables in veterinary medicine. We review the terms commonly used in wearable technology, why it was created, and what role it can play in veterinary medicine to advance care. Although this article is not an exhaustive review of all wearable technology in human or veterinary health care, we will discuss the fundamentals of current technologies (technological advancements) and the philosophies behind how they can benefit veterinary medicine. Finally, we review the adoption barriers, security concerns, and future challenges surrounding wearables.

DEFINITIONS

New technology often comes with intimidating terminology. Although it may be a new vocabulary for veterinarians, and is often outside the scope of traditional veterinary education, practitioners should have a working knowledge of the below definitions to understand how wearables can help them practice medicine now, and in the future.

Artificial Intelligence (AI): Mobile and wearable devices generate an enormous amount of data, and their ability to process this data is beyond a human skill.[3] AI is most often used in combination with a wearable device to digest and extract meaningful knowledge from the data gathered.

Wearable Technology: Wearable technology refers to a type of smart electronic device, which is worn close to the body, which can detect, analyze, and transmit data, and which may include vital signs or environmental data. Wearable technologies, such as the Apple watch (a type of activity tracker), are an example of Internet of Things (IoT). The devices use electronics, software, sensors, and connectivity to exchange data through the Internet with an operator, without requiring any human assistance.[4–6]

Internet of Things: Physical objects that are embedded with sensors that have processing ability, software, and other technologies that connect and exchange data with other devices and systems over the Internet or other communication means.[7–9]

Internet of Medical Things (IoMT), also known as *Smart Health care*: The application of IoT for medical and health-related purposes, data collection, and analysis of research and monitoring. IoMT is the technology used for creating a digitized health-care system that connects available medical resources and health-care services. Examples include remote monitoring devices for tasks such as blood pressure and heart rate, or even something as simple as a smart bed or cage that detects when a patient is occupying it.[10–17]

Internet of Veterinary Things, also known as *Smart Veterinary Health care*: The application of IoT for veterinary health-related purposes.

Epidermal (skin) Electronics: A field of wearable technology termed for its properties and behaviors comparable to those of the epidermis, the outermost layer of skin. Epidermal electronic devices may adhere to the skin via van der Waals forces or elastomeric substrates, and they bend and move with the skin. Often these devices are laminated to the skin. These devices can incorporate electrophysiological, photodetectors, radio frequency inductors, capacitors, oscillators, and rectifying diodes. Solar cells and wireless coils often provide power.[18–20]

Fashion Wearables: Fabrics, garments, and accessories that combine esthetics and style with functional technology.[21]

E-textiles (smart textile or digital textile): The combination of textiles and electronic components to create wearable technology and clothing.[22]

Radiofrequency Identification (RFID): The use of electromagnetic fields to automatically identify and track tags attached to objects. The system consists of a small radio transporter, a radio receiver, and a transmitter. RFID tags can be attached to money, clothing, or implanted in people or animals.

Disruptive Innovation: Innovation that creates a new market and value network and eventually displaces established alliances and cultures.[23] First proposed by Christensen and colleagues, this discovery has led to the Theory of Disruptive Innovations. Disruptive innovations are hallmarked by having initial performance problems that are frustrating to new users.[24,25]

Health care Wearable Device (HWD): A noninvasive medical device that provides a support function or collects data over a prolonged period. This device is typically supported on a part of the human body or the wearer's clothing.[26]

Veterinary Health care Wearable Device (VHWD): A noninvasive medical device that provides a support function or collects data over a prolonged period. This device is typically supported on a part of the animal's body or within a wearable accessory such as a collar or harness.

Bluetooth: A protocol that allows 2 devices to communicate when they are in close proximity.

Near Field Communication (NFC): A set of standards for smart devices to establish radio communication with each other by touching them together or bringing them into proximity, usually no more than a few inches. NFC devices are used in a wide range of applications including payment systems, identification, simple networking, and complex combinations thereof.

Wireless Body Area Networks: Connects independent nodes (eg, sensors and actuators) that are situated in the clothes, on the body, or under the skin of a person. The network typically expands over the whole human body and the nodes are connected through a wireless communication channel.[27]

THE EVOLUTION OF WEARABLES

The concept of a smart device was discussed in 1982, with a modified Coca-Cola vending machine at Carnegie Mellon University. The vending machine was altered to report its inventory and assess if the drinks were cold or not.[28] The notion of the IoT was first conceived by Peter T. Lewis, during his speech to the Congressional Black Caucus Foundation in 1985. He defined IoT as, "the integration of people, processes and technology with connectable devices and sensors to enable remote monitoring, status, manipulation and evaluation of trends of such devices.[29]"

The overall principle of IoT is to embed short-range mobile transceivers in gadgets and daily essentials to enable communication between people and things, and even among things themselves.[30] Cisco Systems later defined IoT in 2011 as "simply the point in time when more 'things or objects' were connected to the Internet than people.[31]"

Since then, IoT has evolved rapidly into the field of IoMT, where wearables are used to collect and analyze data, also known as Smart Health care. The major benefit of IoMT is the creation of a digitized health-care system.[15,16,32] These IoT devices can facilitate remote health monitoring and even emergency notification systems. Devices range from blood pressure and heart rate monitoring to more advanced capabilities such as pacemakers and hearing aids. In 2022, about 25.9% of the human population is a wearables device user.[33]

A 2015 Goldman Sachs report indicates that health-care IoT devices can save the United States more than $300 billion annually in medical expenses by increasing revenue and decreasing cost.[34] Consumers are increasingly adapting and asking for wearable technology. Current research suggests that 80% of consumers are willing to wear an activity monitor.[33] This demand from consumers likely translates to pet owners. The pet wearable market revenue is projected to hit $10 Billion by 2027 and to have a 10.34% CAGR by 2025.[35,36] Pet-specific wearables range from smart harness devices fastened around the pet's body integrated with sensors to monitor a pet's body language, posture and sound, body temperature and heart rate, to smart collars that use GPS, with new technology and products being created each year.

It is also important to state the obvious. As of 2019, 2.5 billion people own a smartphone.[37] There are many sensors readily available on smartphones, including accelerometery, GPS, camera, ambient light, gyroscopes, and microphone detection that can be used as a wearable to monitor people and their pets.[3]

HEALTH CARE WEARABLE DEVICES—WHAT CAN WE LEARN FROM HUMAN MEDICINE?

Remote monitoring, wearables, and their use in telehealth are not new concepts in medicine. Holter monitoring was proposed in the late 1940s as a clinical tool to monitor cardiac arrhythmias at home. Wearable sensors and systems have progressed a great deal since then. These technological tools allow for the early diagnosis of diseases such as congestive heart failure, prevention of diabetes, improved clinical management of neurodegenerative diseases such as Parkinson's, and facilitate the prompt response to emergency situations such as seizures and cardiac arrest.[38] Wearables also have the ability to feed data into an electronic medical record system to facilitate data collection and processing, which can be an important and time-consuming aspect of health care.

Continuous and real-time monitoring of patients with chronic diseases such as diabetes, cardiovascular illness, and neurologic disorders is important. The World Health Organization reports that chronic disease accounts for 75% of all deaths around the world and imposes huge economic burdens on countries, and thus HWDs have the potential to save money and improve care.[39] HWDs can now measure blood pressure, heart rate, ECG, EMG, EEG, EOG, respiratory rate, temperature, blood glucose, blood oxygen levels, and more.[40] Furthermore, point of care wearable devices have changed health care by helping to decrease the load on hospitals by providing more reliable and timely information.[41,42]

CLASSIFICATION OF HEALTH CARE WEARABLE DEVICES

There are several health care wearable devices available, and Iqbal et al. have developed a diagram that can help classify each device (**Figure 1**). Because skin covers most of the human body, it is an ideal place for noninvasive wearable devices. Skin-based wearables can help monitor physiologic and psychological data. They can also be used for the quantitative and qualitative analysis of skin secretions, such as sweat. Skin wearables are either textile based or epidermal based. .

Textile based HWD's can easily monitor temperature, ECG, EEG, or EMG activity. Tattoo or E-skin-based HWDs can be used to monitor ECG, EEG, and EMG. ECG is the easiest to detect because of its high amplitude, which allows for easy detection of heart rhythm through the skin.[43] Luo and colleagues has developed a cuff-less blood pressure measuring device for real-time, continuous measurement of blood pressure using a tattoo-based HWD.[44] It uses a thin flexible piezoelectric sensor with an epidermal ECG sensor for the cuff-less measurement of BP. Other textile based HWDs, such as wearable vests, smart rings, and earphones are available.

One such textile based HWD has been used to detect heart failure, a disease that affects about 26 million people globally.[45] Hafid and colleagues created a wearable

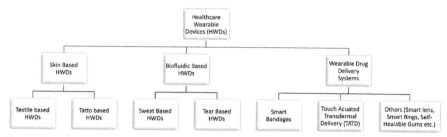

Fig. 1. Classification of Health care Wearable Devices as adopted from Iqbal and colleagues. Iqbal, S.M.A., Mahgoub, I., Du, E. et al. Advances in healthcare wearable devices. npj Flex Electron 5, 9 (2021). https://doi.org/10.1038/s41528-021-00107-x.

system to predict heart failure using variables such as thoracic impedance, heart rate, ECG, and blood oxygen level.[46] Days before heart failure symptoms, such as tachypnea, could be noted fluid is retained in the lungs, which decreases thoracic impedance. The wearable system tracks this information, and alerts when data exceeds the set threshold, identifying heart failure earlier than before. The system transmits a wireless signal over a cloud server to the medical care team.

Some examples include, the Oura metallic ring (Ōura Health Oy. Elektroniikkatie, Finland) that monitors physiologic parameters such as heart rate, body temperature, and breathing. These parameters can be used to monitor for COVID-19.[47–49] The Whoop strap (WHOOP, Boston, Massachusetts) is worn on the wrist, and it collects data such as resting respiratory rate, heart rate, heart rate variability, body temperature, and sleep patterns. This data has been used to help athletes of all levels optimize their health and performance and has also been used in several research studies. Resting respiratory rate data collected by the Whoop strap has been used in a study evaluating whether an individual may be COVID positive 1 to 2 days before the onset of symptoms.[50]

Body secretions such as sweat, saliva, tears, and urine hold important biomarkers. Bio-Fluidic-based HWDs can be used directly or with integration in other platforms. Sen and colleagues have demonstrated the potential to use tears for glucose monitoring.[51] Lin and colleagues have created a smart contact lens for the diagnosis and continuous monitoring of diabetes using tears.[52]

Common variables wearables can measure:

- Heart rate
- Calories burned
- Steps walked
- Blood pressure
- Release of certain biochemicals
- Time spent exercising
- Seizures
- Assessing Mood
- Blood alcohol contents
- Pulse oximetry
- Automatic documentation of care

VETERINARY HEALTH CARE WEARABLE DEVICES

VHWDs are rapidly growing in popularity and can provide veterinary teams with important information. The COVID-19 pandemic has given a swift push to the adoption of technology in veterinary medicine because we have had to learn how to better observe patients from afar and also rely on the owner's description of issues.[53] Global pet wearable market share is mostly identification and tracking, followed by medical diagnosis, safety, and behavior.[54] Lippman describes collars that track a pet's behavior, safety, and health. These can use GPS tracking and the monitoring of resting and sleep patterns, vital signs, as well as licking and scratching behavior. Most wearables on the market today use one or all of the following: RFID, GPS tracking, motion sensors, Bluetooth, accelerometer sensors, and/or cameras/lights.[53]

In an elegant article by Teller and colleagues, high-tech wearables can track activity and provide clues to the early onset of disease. Wearable devices can be attached to an animal's collar and track how active a dog is, how often a cat uses the litterbox, or if pets are drinking more water. We will see the continued development of wearable devices for animals, mobile applications, and data analytics technology that can be developed into a mainstream option.[55]

Additionally, as evidenced by the COVID-19 pandemic in human health care, wearables have a role in disease research, epidemiology, and prevention. Obtaining familiarity with veterinary wearables now can enable us to use them effectively to prevent a similar crisis from happening in animals, especially in herd health settings.

There are numerous benefits to using wearables. Pet owners often are the ones to provide information to veterinarians. However, that information is not always reliable. With wearables, that are appropriately tested and validated, they can produce data that are true and reliable. Information is essential when making an accurate diagnosis and assessing treatment interventions.

Benefits of wearables in veterinary health care:

- Remote monitoring of vital signs
- Pets and owners do not need to travel to send data to a veterinarian
- Improved accessibility of care
- When used appropriately, can support a burdened veterinary care staff
- Facilitate tele-triage
- Monitor postoperative cases
- Support more rapid data gathering
- Monitor animal health in real time
- Diagnoses and treatments begin earlier
- Activity trackers can be beneficial in diagnosing and monitoring multiple diseases
- Collect data for research
- Share and distribute medical information
- Variables that fall outside of set parameters can alert the pet owner or health-care team to an urgent situation
- Engages the pet owner in the health-care team
- Data can be sent to a veterinary specialist for teleconsultation

Wearable data can be helpful to veterinarians in a myriad of ways. Here are select disease examples where wearable data can be transformational in the way medicine is practiced.

- *Pain Management/Arthritis Interventions:* Wearable data can use features that monitor movement to assess how frequently a patient is moving or sleeping. Both dogs and cats may act differently in a veterinary hospital when compared with the at-home setting. Wearables can provide a more accurate understanding of mobility concerns. Chronic conditions such as mobility disorders can be easily tracked and monitored with accelerometers.

- *Cardiovascular and Respiratory Diseases:* Early warning signs that a patient is headed into congestive heart failure or respiratory distress can be tracked with wearables that monitor respiratory rate, heart rate, and pulse oximetry. Telemetry can also be used to assess for the development or progression of arrhythmias.
- *Diabetes:* This disease affects millions of humans around the world. It is a significant area of growth for wearable health-care technology, and the term "diabetes technology" has been coined for devices and software that patients with DM use to aid in their condition.[56] Data has shown that appropriate metabolic control in DM can delay the onset and evolution of its complications.[57] Parameters such as body weight, physical activity, blood pressure, caloric intake, and blood glucose can aid in managing this condition.

Diabetes technologies generally have 2 main categories: those that aid in insulin administration and those that aid in glucose monitoring. Continuous glucose monitors are most often used for monitoring blood glucose levels. More recently, hybrid devices have been developed that do both functions - insulin administration and glucose monitoring. . One large meta-analysis noted that the field of wearable monitoring for DM parameters shows significant promise. Both patients and health-care providers benefit from the easy exchange of data, and because of all the data these devices collect, researchers now have access to data they otherwise would not have.[57]

In veterinary medicine, diabetes is one of the most common diseases in small animal medicine. It is a disease that is often frustrating for the practitioner and owner alike to control. Wearable devices will be the path forward in monitoring and treating these patients because it allows the practitioner to monitor glucose levels and titrate insulin dosing remotely, when the pet is in their own environment.

- *Intraop and Postanesthesia Monitoring:* One of the best ways to decrease anesthesia morbidity and mortality is with the use of technology and appropriate monitoring of vital signs. Wearables allow for the continual stream of data into cloud-based systems, and for automatic alerts to be set when parameters such as pulse oximetry, heart rate, respiratory rate, and temperature fall outside of set parameters. Early recognition and intervention in these settings are critical to providing the best care, and wearables facilitate this.
- *Tele-Triage:* The need for emergency veterinarians continues to outpace supply. Triaging urgent cases is essential for the best medical care. Wearables can stream data into the eyes of veterinarians remotely to assess whether a patient needs to be seen, and if so, how urgent their condition is.
- *Police/Military/Working Dogs:* This segment of the canine population is occasionally challenging to assess and treat due to human safety concerns. Working dogs often have very physically demanding jobs and are prone to injury or distress. The use of wearables facilitates early detection of hyperthermia, and other urgent conditions. Military K9s can be outfitted with wearables that track vital signs and that data can be monitored remotely from a veterinary care team.

CHALLENGES AND FUTURE DIRECTIONS

It is important to know that differences in anatomy, hair type, and skin type can make directly applying existing human technologies to animal species challenging. Often these devices need to be adapted in order to accommodate for anatomic and behavioral differences in veterinary species. Researchers at the Imperial College of London,

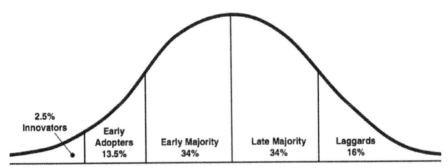

2.5% Innovators

Early Adopters 13.5%

Early Majority 34%

Late Majority 34%

Laggards 16%

Fig. 2. Roger's Diffusion of Innovation Trajectory.[59] From Rogers Everett - Based on Rogers, E. (1962) Diffusion of innovations. Free Press, London, NY, USA. https://en.wikipedia.org/wiki/Diffusion_of_innovations#/media/File:Diffusion_of_ideas.svg.

however, have developed a wearable device that can work through fur.[2] As demand for VHWDs increases from pet owners and veterinarians alike, the technology will continue to blossom and improve as it relates to overcoming the challenges posed by fur, feathers, and scales.

AI will continue to be needed to create filters and algorithms for the extraordinary large data sets that wearables generate. This field is ripe for research and development of AI that can assist the veterinary health-care team more rapidly assess and identify patients that require urgent intervention.

Privacy, autonomy, and control are often concerns that are discussed in human health care because they pertain to wearables and patient data. Although important to consider in veterinary health care, these concerns are often not as high risk as compared with human medicine. Most pet owners seem to willingly share their pet's wearable data. Technology often develops first, and then privacy, autonomy, and control concerns are identified after the fact, when the wearable is deployed on a larger scale. For this reason, veterinary professionals need to continue to be vigilant about the privacy of a patient's data.

BARRIERS TO ADOPTION

Wearable technology has the ability to profoundly advance veterinary health care. However, we are still at the "early adoption" stage of Everett Roger's diffusion of innovation trajectory (**Figure 2**). This diffusion is a process by which innovation is communicated through various channels over time, among members of a social system. These channels are often relationships built between 2 individuals, and based on interpersonal relationships. Innovation is first adopted by the people who created it. Later, it goes through a cycle of adoption, culminating with standardization and mainstream acceptance.[58] This process can take a significant amount of time.

Although health-care systems are often reluctant to change, there is optimism surrounding how quickly veterinary medicine can adopt wearables. This is because these devices offer several benefits including: enhanced connectivity, improved usability, reduced cost, increased reliability, and long battery life, and they are well proven in human medicine.[1] The authors encourage all veterinarians to be open minded to using and experimenting with wearable devices in their practice .

SUMMARY

A new era of interaction among people, pets, vets, and technology is starting. The wearable revolution is coming to a veterinary practice near you. As the technology becomes increasingly more affordable and accessible, and connects with cloud-based systems already used in veterinary health ecosystems, we will see exponential growth in this market. The benefits of using wearables in veterinary health care are immense. Wearables can make our veterinary health-care systems more accessible, efficient, and responsive to patient and owner needs. This leads to enhanced care and earlier recognition of disease.

DISCLOSURE

A. Mitek and S. Vitale are cofounders of Stratocyte, a virtual marketplace that connects veterinary specialists with primary care veterinarians around the world. A. Mitek is owner of AnesthesiaDiva.com, and provides anesthesia teleconsultations and training to veterinary healthcare providers globally. A. Newell and D. Jones are cofounders of Animal Cloud Device Connectivity, Inc., a cloud-based software company that leverages the power of military grade technology to monitor and maintain an animal's medical record and vital signs.

REFERENCES

1. Sultan N. Reflective thoughts on the potential and challenges of wearable technology for healthcare provision and medical education. Int J Inf Management 2015;35(5):521–6.
2. Andreu-Perez J, et al, Andreu-Perez, Javier, Daniel R. Leff, Henry MD Ip, and Guang-Zhong Yang. From wearable sensors to smart implants—toward pervasive and personalized healthcare. IEEE Trans Biomed Eng 2015;62(12):2750–62.
3. Banos O, Villalonga C, Bang J, et al. Human Behavior Analysis by Means of Multimodal Context Mining. Sensors (Basel) 2016;16(8):1264.
4. Libra use in dogs and cats. Available at: https://veterinarypartner.vin.com/default.aspx?pid=19239&id=9150771. Accessed December 20, 2021.
5. Continuous Glucose Monitoring in Veterinary Patients. Available at: https://todaysveterinarypractice.com/continuous-glucose-monitoring-in-veterinary-patients/. Accessed December 20, 2021.
6. Düking P, Achtzehn S, Holmberg HC, et al. Integrated Framework of Load Monitoring by a Combination of Smartphone Applications, Wearables and Point-of-Care Testing Provides Feedback that Allows Individual Responsive Adjustments to Activities of Daily Living. Sensors (Basel) 2018;18(5). https://doi.org/10.3390/s18051632.
7. Düking P, Hotho A, Holmberg HC, et al. Comparison of Non-Invasive Individual Monitoring of the Training and Health of Athletes with Commercially Available Wearable Technologies. Front Physiol 2016;7:71.
8. O'Donoghue J, Herbert J. Data Management Within mHealth Environments: Patient Sensors, Mobile Devices, and Databases. J Data Inf Qual 2012;4(1). 5: 1–5:20.
9. Gillis, Alexander (2021). "What is internet of things (IoT)?". IOT Agenda. Retrieved 17 August 2021.
10. da Costa CA, Pasluosta CF, Eskofier B, et al. Internet of Health Things: Toward intelligent vital signs monitoring in hospital wards. Artif Intelligence Med 2018; 89:61–9.

11. Engineer A, Sternberg EM, Najafi B. Designing Interiors to Mitigate Physical and Cognitive Deficits Related to Aging and to Promote Longevity in Older Adults: A Review. Gerontology 2018;64(6):612–22.

12. Kricka LJ. History of disruptions in laboratory medicine: what have we learned from predictions? Clin Chem Lab Med 2019;57(3):308–11.

13. Gatouillat A, Badr Y, Massot B, et al. Internet of Medical Things: A Review of Recent Contributions Dealing with Cyber-Physical Systems in Medicine"(PDF). IEEE Internet Things J 2018;5(5):3810–22.

14. Topol E. The patient will see you now: the future of medicine is in your hands, . New York, New York. Basic Books; 2016.

15. Dey N, Hassanien AE, Bhatt C, et al. Internet of things and big data analytics toward next-generation intelligence(PDF). New York, NY. Springer International Publishing; 2018. Retrieved 14 October 2018.

16. Pratap Singh R, Javaid M, Haleem A, et al. Internet of Medical Things (IoMT) for orthopaedic in COVID-19 pandemic: Roles, challenges, and applications. J Clin Orthop Trauma 2020;11(4):713–7.

17. "Deloitte Centre for Health Solutions" (PDF). Deloitte. Available at: https://www2.deloitte.com/content/dam/Deloitte/uk/Documents/life-sciences-health-care/deloitte-uk-connected-health.pdf. Accessed December 20, 2021.

18. Kim D-H, Rogers J. Epidermal Electronics. Science 2011;333(6044):838–43. Bibcode:2011Sci...333..838K.

19. Webb RC, Ma Y, Krishnan S, et al. Epidermal devices for noninvasive, precise, and continuous mapping of macrovascular and microvascular blood flow. Sci Adv 2015;1(9):e1500701. Bibcode:2015SciA....1E0701W.

20. Zhang, Y; Tao, TH. (2019). "Skin-Friendly Electronics for Acquiring Human Physiological Signatures". Adv Mater. 31 (49): 1905767.

21. Seymour S. Fashionable Technology: the intersection of design, fashion, science and technology. New York: Springer Wien; 2008.

22. E-Textiles 2019-2029: Technologies, Markets and Players: IDTechEx. 2019. Available at: www.idtechex.com.

23. Ab Rahman, Airini; et al. (2017). "Emerging Technologies with Disruptive Effects: A Review". PERINTIS eJournal. 7 (2). Retrieved 21 December 2017.

24. Christensen CM. The innovator's dilemma: when new technologies cause great firms to fail. Harvard Business Review Press; 2013.

25. Christensen C, Raynor M. The innovator's solution: creating and sustaining successful growth. Brighton, Massachusetts. Harvard Business Review Press; 2013.

26. D. Hemapriya, P. Viswanath, V. M. Mithra, S. Nagalakshmi and G. Umarani, "Wearable medical devices — Design challenges and issues," 2017 International Conference on Innovations in Green Energy and Healthcare Technologies (IGEHT), 2017, pp. 1-6, doi: 10.1109/IGEHT.2017.8094096.

27. Wireless Body Area Networks. Ghent University. Available at: https://www.waves.intec.ugent.be/research/wireless-body-area-networks. Accessed January 15, 2021.

28. Teicher Jordan, IBM. Website. https://www.ibm.com/blogs/industries/little-known-story-first-iot-device/. Accessed December 20, 2021.. The little known story of the first IoT device, 10 IBM; 2018. February 2018.

29. Sharma, Chetan. "Correcting the IoT History". Chetan Sharma Blog. 14 March 2016. Retrieved 1 June 2021.

30. Stallings W. Foundations of modern networking : SDN, NFV, QoE, IoT, and cloud. Indianapolis, Indiana: Florence Agboma, Sofiene Jelassi; 2016. OCLC 927715441.

31. Dave Evans (April 2011). "The Internet of Things: How the Next Evolution of the Internet Is Changing Everything" (PDF). CISCO White Paper and Website.

32. Deloitte Centre for. Health Solutions. Deloitte website. https://www2.deloitte.com/us/en/pages/life-sciences-and-health-care/topics/center-for-health-solutions.html.

33. Phaneuf, Alicia. Latest trends in medical monitoring devices and wearable health technology. 1/22/21. Available at: https://www.businessinsider.com/wearable-technology-healthcare-medical-devices. Accessed December 20, 2021.

34. Barksdale Matthew. "Goldman Sachs report: how the internet of things can save the American healthcare system $305 billion annually". Engage mobile blog. LinkedIn. Engage Mobile Solutions, LLC; 2016. Retrieved 26 July 2018.

35. Global Market Insights Inc. Pet Wearable Market revenue to hit $10 Bn by 2027. Available at: https://www.globenewswire.com/en/news-release/2021/06/03/2240977/0/en/Pet-Wearable-Market-revenue-to-hit-10-Bn-by-2027-Global-Market-Insights-Inc.html. Accessed December 20, 2021.

36. Opportunities in the World Market for Pet Wearables to 2025: Growth in Demand for Pet Monitoring with Identification and Tracking Segment Set for a CAGR of 10.34%. 10/20/2020. Available at: https://www.globenewswire.com/news-release/2020/10/20/2111298/28124/en/Opportunities-in-the-World-Market-for-Pet-Wearables-to-2025-Growth-in-Demand-for-Pet-Monitoring-with-Identification-and-Tracking-Segment-Set-for-a-CAGR-of-10-34.html. Accessed December 20, 2021.

37. Demographics of mobile device ownership and adoption in the United States. Pew Research Center. [2019-06-24]. Available at: https://www.pewinternet.org/fact-sheet/mobile/. Accessed December 20, 2021.

38. Bonato, Paolo. "Advances in wearable technology and its medical applications." 2010 annual international conference of the IEEE engineering in medicine and biology. IEEE, 2010.

39. Amine EK, et al, Who, J., & Consultation, F. E. (2003). Diet, nutrition and the prevention of chronic diseases. World Health Organ Tech Rep Ser, 916(i-viii), 1-149.. Diet, nutrition and the prevention of chronic diseases. World Health Organ Tech Rep Ser 2003. https://doi.org/10.1093/ajcn/60.4.644a.

40. Iqbal SMA, Mahgoub I, Du E, et al. Advances in healthcare wearable devices. Npj Flex Electron 2021;5:9.

41. Bhalla N, Jolly P, Formisano N, et al. Introduction to biosensors. Essays Biochem 2016;60:1–8.

42. Kim J, Campbell AS, de Ávila BEF, et al. Wearable biosensors for healthcare monitoring. Nat. Biotechnol 2019;37:389–406.

43. Someya T, Amagai M. Toward a new generation of smart skins. Nat Biotechnol 2019;37:382–8.

44. Luo N, et al, Luo, Ningqi, Wenxuan Dai, Chenglin Li, Zhiqiang Zhou, Liyuan Lu, Carmen CY Poon, Shih-Chi Chen, Yuanting Zhang, and Ni Zhao. Flexible piezoresistive sensor patch enabling ultralow power cuffless blood pressure measurement. Adv Funct Mater 2016;26:1178–87.

45. Savarese G, Lund LH. Pharmacological therapy nitrates as a treatment of acute heart failure pharmacological therapy. J Hear Team 2016;3:51–5.

46. Hafid A, et al, Hafid, Abdelakram, Sara Benouar, Malika Kedir-Talha, Farhad Abtahi, Mokhtar Attari, and Fernando Seoane. Full impedance cardiography measurement device using raspberry PI3 and system-on-chip biomedical instrumentation solutions. IEEE J Biomed Heal Inform 2018;22:1883–94.

47. Yan Z. Unprecedented pandemic, unprecedented shift, and unprecedented opportunity. Hum Behav Emerg Technol 2020;2:110–2.

48. Chicago "The species Severe acute respiratory syndrome-related coronavirus: classifying 2019-nCoV and naming it SARS-CoV-2." Nature microbiology 5, no. 4 (2020): 536-544.. The species Severe acute respiratory syndrome-related coronavirus: classifying 2019-nCoV and naming it SARS-CoV-2. Nat Microbiol 2020;5: 536–44.

49. Kabir MA, et al, Kabir, MD Alamgir, Rajib Ahmed, Sheikh Muhammad Asher Iqbal, Rasheduzzaman Chowdhury, Ramasamy Paulmurugan, Utkan Demirci, and Waseem Asghar.. Diagnosis for COVID-19: current status and future prospects. Expert Rev Mol Diagn 2021. https://doi.org/10.1080/14737159.2021.1894930.

50. Natarajan A, Su HW, Heneghan C, et al. Measurement of respiratory rate using wearable devices and applications to COVID-19 detection. Npj Digit Med 2021;4:136.

51. Sen DK, Sarin GS. Tear glucose levels in normal people and in diabetic patients. Br J Ophthalmol 1980;64:693–5.

52. Lin YR, et al, Lin, You-Rong, Chin-Chi Hung, Hsien-Yi Chiu, Po-Han Chang, Bor-Ran Li, Sheng-Jen Cheng, Jia-Wei Yang, Shien-Fong Lin, and Guan-Yu Chen.. Noninvasive glucose monitoring with a contact lens and smartphone. Sensors 2018;18:1–12.

53. The latest on pet wearables. DVM 360. Available at: https://www.dvm360.com/view/the-latest-on-pet-wearables. Accessed December 20, 2021.

54. Global pet wearable market by share. Available at: https://www.softeq.com/blog/iot-wearables-keep-pets-healthy-happy-and-safe-why-and-how. Accessed December 20, 2021.

55. Teller, Lori Massin, and Heather K. Moberly. "Veterinary Telemedicine: A literature review." Veterinary Evidence article (2020).

56. Rodriguez-León C, Villalonga C, Munoz-Torres M, et al. Mobile and Wearable Technology for the Monitoring of Diabetes-Related Parameters: Systematic Review. JMIR Mhealth Uhealth 2021;9(6):e25138.

57. Diabetes. World Health Organization. [2020-07-24]. Available at: https://www.who.int/diabetes/action_online/basics/en/index3.html. Accessed December 20, 2021.

58. Rogers EM. Diffusion of innovations. 3rd edition. New York: Free Press; 1983.

59. Rogers Everett - Based on Rogers E. Diffusion of innovations. London: Free Press; 1962. Available at: https://en.wikipedia.org/wiki/Diffusion_of_innovations#/media/File:Diffusion_of_ideas.svg.

Anesthesiologists in the Ether

Technology and Telemedicine in Anesthesiology

Ashley Mitek, DVM, MS, DACVAA

KEYWORDS

- Telehealth • Telemedicine • Anesthesiology • Artificial intelligence • Teleconsulting
- Remote anesthetic monitoring • Electronic anesthesia medical record
- Anesthesia information management system

KEY POINTS

- Veterinary anesthesiologists can now provide synchronous and asynchronous teleconsulting services to primary care practitioners.
- Veterinary hospitals should consider transitioning to an electronic anesthesia record system because they enhance patient care and minimize human error.
- Artificial Intelligence will impact many aspects of veterinary anesthesiology for the better.
- In the coming decade, there will be an alternative care model available for veterinary anesthesiologists that enables them to remotely monitor patients and consult with medical teams from afar using cloud-based healthcare communication solutions.

TELEMEDICINE AND ANESTHESIA
Introduction

Anesthesia depends on technology. The 2 fields are inseparable. Perhaps the greatest benefit of the advancing technology has been the drastic decrease in morbidity and mortality rates. Information is essential. Technology helps one more efficiently gather this information to make the best anesthetic decision. Technology has also facilitated the expansion of anesthesiology into the realm of telehealth. Ten years ago, it would have been unheard of for a veterinary anesthesiologist to work remotely. But today, that care model is changing, and anesthesiologists can share their knowledge far beyond the confines of an operating room.

For instance, preoperative anesthetic evaluations can easily be performed via synchronous or asynchronous teleconsultations. The same goes for intraoperative, and postoperative care. In addition, patient health-related anesthetic data can be accessed remotely by an anesthesiologist with the click of a button. This article

Co-Founder, Stratocyte.com, Owner, AnesthesiaDiva.com, 48-113 Angel Wing PeakGlacier National Park, MT, USA
E-mail address: diva@anesthesiadiva.com

Vet Clin Small Anim 52 (2022) 1099–1107
https://doi.org/10.1016/j.cvsm.2022.06.002
0195-5616/22/© 2022 Elsevier Inc. All rights reserved.

reviews a select number of advances in anesthesiology relating to telemedicine, including automation, artificial intelligence, and remote monitoring . Also covered is the new care model of anesthesiologists working in telehealth. Advancing technology and telehealth hold exciting opportunities for addressing the current shortage of veterinary anesthesiologists, and have the potential to make care more equitable and accessible to the patients who need it most.

Definitions

The anesthesia electronic medical record (AEMR) is an electronic system that captures clinical anesthesia patient data.[1,2] In human medicine, the AEMR has become more specialized and automated into an AIMS.

Anesthesia information management systems (AIMS) are specialized AEMR networks that improve patient safety, operations management, billing, and research.[2–4]

Artificial intelligence is the study of algorithms that give machines the ability to reason and perform functions such as problem solving, object and word recognition, inference of world states, and decision making.[5,6]

Synchronous (real-time) anesthesia teleconsulting (SAT) occurs when a veterinarian or technician interact with an anesthesiologist by phone or video conference. Text or chat-based synchronous teleconsulting is also possible, but used less frequently. SAT is ideally suited for urgent case consultations.

Asynchronous (store and forward) anesthesia teleconsulting (AAT) is the practice by which a veterinarian or technician communicates with an anesthesiologist by text or chat feature. This system is ideal for nonurgent anesthesia questions, and in some situations it can be converted to a SAT if needed.

Remote patient monitoring (RPM) is the ability to capture and electronically transmit patient physiologic data to healthcare providers.

Anesthesia Electronic Medical Records

Many veterinary hospitals are currently transitioning to an AEMR, because they have many benefits to the patient, the provider and the overall health care ecosystem. Paper anesthesia records were initially created in the 1890s.[7,8] Pulse, temperature, and respiratory rate were the initial variables that were documented. In 1902, blood pressure measurement was incorporated.[9] Today, veterinary providers typically have many more variables on an anesthesia record, including, pulse oximetry, capnography, ventilation data, volatile anesthetic concentration, drugs and doses utilized, and patient-specific notes in addition to other items.

The next logical progression of a paper record would be manual entry of data into a computer and then automated capture of data. Automated capture of physiologic data was first described in the 1930s, and early attempts at this occurred in the 1970s.[10] But we did not see a complete transition in human medicine from paper to electronic until more recently.[11–13] Initially these records were homegrown local hospital applications, before AIMS was discussed at the American Society of Anesthesiologists annual meeting in 1989.[11,14–16] When these electronic systems were initially created, there was sluggish adoption of the technology, as is typical with innovation.

Automated anesthesia EMRs were initially developed to capture data. They have been shown to have many benefits.[10] The Anesthesia Patient Safety Foundation (APSF) has strongly voiced that it "endorse(s) and advocate(s) the use of automated record keeping in the perioperative period and the subsequent retrieval and analysis of the data to improve patient safety."[17] Although many providers are resistant to convert from paper records to electronic, it is now best practice to utilize electronic records, and all practices should consider implementing this software, because it provides for the best patient care.

There is a steep learning curve when initially converting from paper to electronic records, and a tablet is needed for all staff performing anesthesia. This challenge is usually surmounted by decreasing case load for the first one-two weeks the software is rolled out. In addition, it is ideal to train staff ahead of time on the new software, and ensure adequate technological support is available on-site when the software is deployed.

Anesthesia providers can have tremendous cognitive loads when working with a patient. Providers are often multitasking, setting up equipment, monitoring the patient, and making a written anesthesia record. By using electronic records, the provider's cognitive load is decreased , allowing the provider to focus attention on the patient.

Electronic records also allow anesthesia providers to gain easy access to patient information. That is because the AEMR can be connected to the electronic medical record for seamless integration. Hand-written anesthesia records are also notoriously illegible. Electronic records still allow a provider to input manual notes about a patient, but all data are legible. AEMR can also help patients have an overall positive anesthetic experience, because they allow the provider to quickly view his or her past anesthesia records. Furthermore, they can generate significant data for analytics and research, and help practices recognize areas for improvement.

Benefits of AEMR[7,10] include

1. Reducing the anesthesia provider cognitive load
2. Facilitating situational awareness and point of care clinical decision making
3. Easy access to patient information
4. Creating a legible anesthetic record
5. Easily viewing past patient history
6. Generating significant data for analytics
7. Interfacing with billing software
8. Eliminating recall bias
9. Protocol compliance
10. Can help guide users through airway management or cardiopulmonary resuscitation (CPR) situations
11. Supporting quality improvement and research
12. All-in-one library of drugs, dosages, and reference guides
13. Customized drugs for CPR and other common conditions
14. Minimizing calculation errors

Anesthesia Information Management Systems

AIMS are specialized EMRs that interface with hospital clinical data repositories and provide users with access to patient data, including laboratory, billing, imaging, pharmacy, and other aspects of the health record. AIMS can automatically pull in vital signs from monitoring devices and anesthesia machines, for example.[2–4,7] AIMS are the future of veterinary anesthesiology. They are also beneficial to anesthesiologists who provide telehealth services, because they allow the specialist to access all of the patient's records in 1 location.

Limitations of Electronic Anesthesia Records

Electronic anesthesia records have many benefits. However, there are still limitations to their use in practice. Artifactual readings can sometimes occur, and the philosophy of garbage in, garbage out applies.[3,18] It is imperative that equipment is attached to the patient correctly and that staff members on site are trained to use that equipment and identify artifactual readings. Most technology in electronic anesthesia records needs a network connection, and if that connection fails, the software and/or hardware may not work appropriately.[19] A power supply, or ability to charge a battery, is an obvious need for tablets and other devices. Although rare, cyberattacks have been identified as a concern, and electronic anesthesia records have been noted to be more beneficial in malpractice defense in human anesthesia,.[2–4,18,20] Veterinary anesthesia poses specific unique concerns when transitioning to electronic records, because there is no standardized system for monitoring anesthetized patients. This has led to varying standards and minimal regulation surrounding the use and the adoption of electronic anesthesia records in veterinary practice.

It should also be noted that transitioning from a paper anesthetic record to an electronic one can be expensive. Many hospitals have found this transition to be beneficial, and to be a great return on investment. The other downside to EMR is that staff need to be trained appropriately to use the system, and this typically requires 1-2 weeks of reduced service to facilitate learning and adoption of the new technology. Technological support staff are also ideal to have on-site or at least available remotely to triage urgent technological problems.

Anesthesia Telemedicine and Teleconsulting

Traditionally, anesthesiologists in both the human and veterinary health care ecosystems were clinicians who lived in operating rooms. The notion of an anesthesiologist being valuable outside the confines of a brick and mortar hospital were not possible. However, with the advent of new technology, as long as one has appropriately trained staff to administer anesthesia in an operating room, and equipment to acquire physiologic data, an anesthesiologist can consult on cases anywhere in the world.

Asynchronous Anesthesia Teleconsulting

Asynchronous teleconsulting is when an anesthesiologist interacts with a care provider in a manner that is not time dependent . Chat-based teleconsulting platforms work great for this, and email can also work, although it can be challenging to incorporate into the pateint's electronic medical record. Arguably, there are always times where it is ideal to have an anesthesiologist in an operating room. However, a new model is emerging to combat the relative shortage of veterinary anesthesiologists compared with the overwhelming demand. There are many ways that anesthesiologists can be helpful remotely. One method is for an anesthesiologist to assist with a preoperative consultation. A technician or veterinarian on site can work-up a case, and then discuss the concerns about the patient and procedure with an anesthesiologist via phone, video, or chat. This streamlines the delivery of expertise and knowledge.

This model of teleconsultations aligns with Adam Smith's philosophy on division of labor.[21] If individuals are allowed to specialize in the care they can provide, efficiencies can be enhanced and better overall care provided. By having a technician, veterinarian, or robot on site assess, work-up, and physically deliver anesthesia care, the anesthesiologist can be free to help with many cases simultaneously from anywhere in the world.

Synchronous Anesthesia Teleconsulting

Remote anesthesiologists can provide real-time or stat recommendations in operating rooms with the use of traditional audio, video, and chat connections. The future of anesthesiology will likely trend toward what has happened in the field of veterinary radiology. An anesthesiologist may soon be sitting behind several computer monitors, similar to a "reading room" radiologists were accustomed to in the past. This setup can be physically deployed in a room within the confines of a hospital, or in a remote location. Smartphones, tablets and laptops can also be used when anesthesiologists are on the go. Regardless of the device used, the screen showcases patient data from any anesthetized patient around the world. Technicians and veterinarians on site will deliver the anesthesia, and the remote anesthesiologist will be available for more complex matters in asynchronous and synchronous communication platforms.

This type of system has already been used successfully by the US military. BATDOK is a multipatient, point of injury, casualty tool that allows medics on the ground to collect vital patient data and stream them to clinicians and specialists at remote locations (**Fig. 1**).[22] A medic can place a sensor like a pulse oximeter, or blood pressure device on a patient, and the sensor will automatically start recording without even having to open the application on a smartphone. This allows the medic to focus on the patient instead of focusing on writing down data points. In addition, BATDOK is an advantageous system because of its open architecture. It can be easily updated and adapt to new hardware.[22] Expert clinicians not present on the battle ground can then see patient data and help medics treat a case. This is an example of remote patient monitoring (RPM), which will be increasingly more common in both human and veterinary anesthesia.

Another new piece of technology that can facilitate anesthesia teleconsultations is from a company called VetMeasure, which has released a wearable called MeasureON!. The device incorporates sensors into a harness that collects ECG, temperature, respiratory rate, heart rate, environmental temperature, environmental humidity, and activity level data. Although a comprehensive review on wearables is outside the scope of this article, this is an example of a device that can automatically capture important patient vital signs and relay them to a cloud for an anesthesiologist to view remotely.[23]

Benefits of anesthesia teleconsulting[24] include

- Increasing access to specialty consultations in underserved populations
- Remote preoperative, intraoperative, and postoperative advice can be provided
- Teleconsulting may decrease the cost of care, as well as morbidity and mortality rates
- Allows an anesthesiologist to assist with multiple patients simultaneously

Artificial Intelligence

In the past decade, artificial intelligence has significantly advanced the field of anesthesiology.[6] In an article by Hashimoto and colleagues,[6] the authors describe 6

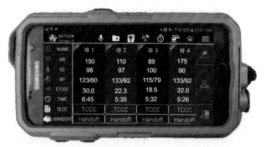

Fig. 1. BATDOK software showcasing 4 different patient parameters relaying into a smartphone so a clinician can monitor and assist with multiple patients. (U.S Air Force.)

domains where AI has emerged in the field: depth of anesthetic monitoring, control of anesthesia, event and risk prediction, ultrasound guidance, pain management, and operating room logistics. One definition of artificial intelligence is the study of algorithms that give machines the ability to reason and perform functions such as problem solving, object and word recognition, inference of world states, and decision making.[5] In April 2018, the US Food and Drug Administration approved the first software system that uses artificial intelligence to assist in the diagnosis of diabetic retinopathy by analyzing images of the fundus.[25] The important word here is *assist*. Artificial intelligence will not replace anesthesiologists, but it will significantly help them in the near future make the best decisions for patients. A deep dive into the future of artificial intelligence in veterinary anesthesiology is outside the scope of this article. However, technology, including artificial intelligence, can facilitate anesthesiologists consulting on cases around the world by helping to filter the raw data that are acquired on-site, and sending those data to the anesthesiologist for review and further assessment.

Tools Versus Machines and Automation

A tool is powered directly by its user, and a machine augments its user's input using external power, but remains directly under the user's control.[26] Seger and colleagues explain that automation is the ability of a machine to alter its function without direct user input, but in pursuit of a user-defined objective. In the past, anesthesiologists have mostly used tools and machines. But automation is changing that. Closed-loop anesthesia systems (CLADS) have a closed feedback loop and are like cruise control in a car. A ventilator can be trained to reach a certain goal (such as end-tidal carbon dioxide), and be in control of an input that affects that goal (such as minute ventilation).[26] CLADS controlled total intravenous anesthesia infusions have been shown to more tightly regulate anesthetic depth, shorten recovery time, and reduce sedative agent consumption.[27]

In an editorial entitled "Robots will Perform Anesthesia in The Near Future" in *Anesthesiology*, the author discusses the way that automation will change the way anesthesia is delivered.[28] Many studies have found that automated anesthesia systems outperform controls.[29,30] This automation will trickle into veterinary anesthesia over the next 10 years. These advances will impact how an anesthesiologist functions on a daily basis. Instead of physically being in an operating room, it may be a better use of an anesthesiologist's time to remotely consult on cases, or sit in a "Reading Room" within a hospital where patient vital signs are streamed in on multiple screens. On-site health care team members and robots may actually perform the anesthesia, but they will not replace the need for an anesthesiologist. In fact, improving technology and artificial intelligence will facilitate the collection of more complex data that require the training and experience of an anesthesiologist to best process them. Advancing technology is only going to increase the demand for anesthesiologists in veterinary medicine.

Reduction of Human Error

To err is human

—Alexander Pope

People make mistakes. Various factors lead people to err in their medical decision making, such as sleep deprivation, missing data, lack of appropriate experience or training, and other environmental factors. Most adverse anesthetic events can be traced back to a human error.[31,32] Many anesthesiologists cite that advances in anesthesia technology and monitoring have profoundly reduced morbidity and mortality rates.[33] With the invention and adoption of new technology, it is likely that morbidity and mortality rates will continue to decrease. Information is essential. Artificial intelligence algorithms will identify problems before the human eye or brain can identify them, and can alert team members at on-site locations and remote teleconsulting anesthesiologists of a patient's potential declining condition. Primary care clinicians and anesthesiologists alike should be optimistic about the future of incorporating anesthesia teleconsulting into day-to-day primary care practice as needed for complex cases.

SUMMARY

A new frontier is emerging in veterinary anesthesiology. Anesthesiologists have traditionally been accessible only to those patients who come to a university teaching hospital, or a tertiary care facility. However, with the enhanced adoption of electronic anesthesia recording systems and teleconsulting technology anesthesiologists will be able to positively impact underserved patients around the world.

CLINICS CARE POINTS

- Research in human medicine has repeatedly shown that electronic anesthesia records lead to better patient outcomes.
- Primary care veterinarians around the world can now obtain a virtual anesthesia or pain management consultation (synchronous or asynchronous) from an anesthesiologist.
- Studies have repeatedly demonstrated that automated anesthesia systems and advancing technology significantly reduces morbidity and mortality in humans.

DISCLOSURES

A. Mitek is cofounder of Stratocyte.com, a virtual marketplace that connects veterinary specialists with primary care veterinarians around the world. She also owns AnesthesiaDiva.com, and provides anesthesia teleconsultations and training to veterinary healthcare providers globally. A. Mitek has a working relationship with Animal Device Connectivity, INC, a company that has licensed BATDOK software from the United States Air Force.

REFERENCES

1. Egger Halbeis CB, et al, Halbeis, Christoph B. Egger, Richard H. Epstein, Alex Macario, Ronald G. Pearl, and Zvi Grunwald. Adoption of anesthesia information management systems by academic departments in the United States. Anesth Analg 2008;107(4):1323–9.
2. Ehrenfeld JM, Rehman MA. Anesthesia information management systems: a review of functionality and installation considerations. J Clin Monit Comput 2011; 25(1):71–9.
3. Epstein RH, Dexter F. Database quality and access issues relevant to research using anesthesia information management system data. Anesth Analg 2018; 127(1):105–14.
4. Gage JS, et al, Gage, J. S., S. Subramanian, J. F. Dydro, and P. J. Poppers. "Automated anesthesia surgery medical record system." International journal of

clinical monitoring and computing 7, no. 4 (1990): 259-263. Automated anesthesia surgery medical record system. Int J Clin Monit Comput 1990;7(4):259–63.

5. Bellman R. An introduction to artificial intelligence: can computers think? San Francisco: Boyd & Fraser Pub Co; 1978.

6. Hashimoto DA, Witkowski E, Gao L, et al. Artificial intelligence in anesthesiology: current techniques, clinical applications, and limitations. Anesthesiology 2020; 132:379–94.

7. Rozental O, White RS. Anesthesia information management systems: evolution of the paper anesthetic record to a multisystem electronic medical record network that streamlines perioperative care. J Anesth Hist 2019;3:93–8.

8. Kadry, et al, Kadry, Bassam, William W. Feaster, Alex Macario, and Jesse M. Ehrenfeld. Anesthesia information management systems: past, present, and future of anesthesia records. Mt Sinai J Med 2012;79(1):154–65.

9. Fisher JA, Bromberg IL, Eisen LB. On the design of anaesthesia record forms. Can J Anaesth 1994;41(10):973–83.

10. Cordtz C. Five Benefits of Electronic Anesthesia Record Software. March 19, 2020. Surgical Information Systems. Available at: https://blog.sisfirst.com/5-benefits-of-electronic-anesthesia-record-software. Accessed 1.1.2022.

11. E.G. Hoffner, Anesthesia Information Management Systems: A Review of the History, Products, and the Adoption of Systems. (2013).

12. McKesson EI. The technique of recording the effects of gas-oxygen mixtures, pressures, rebreathing and carbon-dioxide, with a summary of the effects. Curr Res Anesth Analg 1934;13:1–7.

13. Shah NJ, Tremper KK, Kheterpal S. Anatomy of an anesthesia information management system. Anesthesiol Clin 2011;29(3):355–65.

14. Wang X, Gardner RM, Seager PR. Integrating computerized anesthesia charting into a hospital information system. Int J Clin Monit Comput 1995;12(2):61–70.

15. Abenstein JP, et al, Abenstein, J. P., C. B. DeVos, and S. Tarhan. "Eight year's experience with automated anesthesia record keeping: lessons learned—new directions taken." International journal of clinical monitoring and computing 9, no. 2 (1992): 117-129. Eight year's experience with automated anesthesia record keeping: lessons learned—new directions taken. Int J Clin Monit Comput 1992;9(2): 117–29.

16. Eichhorm JH, Edsall DW. Computerization of anesthesia information management. J Clin Monit 1991;7(1):71–82.

17. Anesthesia Patient Safety Foundation. Anesthesia Patient Safety Foundation Newsletter. 2001. Available at:http://www.apsf.org/newsletters/html/2001/winter/02ARK.htm. .

18. Liem VGB, et al, Liem, Victor GB, Sanne E. Hoeks, Felix van Lier, and Jurgen C. de Graaff. What we can learn from big data about factors influencing perioperative outcome. Curr Opin Anaesthesiol 2018;31(6):723–31.

19. Vakharia SB, Rinehart J. Using anesthesia AIMS data in quality management. Int Anesthesiol Clin 2014;52(1):42–52.

20. Stol IS, Ehrenfeld JM, Epstein RH. Technology diffusion of anesthesia information management systems into academic anesthesia departments in the. United StatesAnesth Analg 2014;118(3):644–50.

21. Smith AM. Wealth of nations. Oxford: England: Bibliomania; 2002.

22. Bedi Shireen. Batdok Improves, tailors to deployment. Air Force Surgeon General Public Affairs 2019.

23. VetMeasure. Available at: https://vetmeasure.com. Accessed on 1/1/2022.

24. Chatrath V, Pal Attri J, Raman C. Telemedicine and anaesthesia. Indian J Anaesthesia 2010;3:199.
25. FDA. FDA permits marketing of artificial intelligence-based device to detect certain diabetes-related eye problems. FDA US Food and Drug Administration; 2018.
26. Seger CN, Cannesson M. Recent advances in the technology of anesthesia. F1000Research 2020.
27. Pasin L, Nardelli P, Pintaudi M, et al. Closed-loop delivery systems versus manually controlled administration of total IV anesthesia: a meta-analysis of randomized clinical trials. Anesth Analg 2017;124(2):456–64.
28. Robots will perform anesthesia in the near future. Hemmerling TM Anesthesiology 2020;132(2):219–20.
29. Joosten A, Rinehart J, Bardaji A, et al. Anesthetic management using multiple closed-loop systems and delayed neurocognitive recovery: a randomized controlled trial. Anesthesiology 2020;132:253–66.
30. Brogi E, Cyr S, Kazan R, et al. Clinical performance and safety of closed-loop systems: a systematic review and meta-analysis of randomized controlled trials. Anesth Analg 2017;124:446–55.
31. Merry AF, Webster CS. Has anesthesia care become safer and is anesthesia-related mortality decreasing? F1000 Med Rep 2009;1:69.
32. Webb RK, Currie M, Morgan CA, et al. The Australian Incident Monitoring Study: an analysis of 2000 incident reports. Anaesth Intensive Care 1993;21:520–8.
33. Chilkoti G, Wadhwa R, Saxena AK. Technological advances in perioperative monitoring: current concepts and clinical perspectives. J Anaesthesiol Clin Pharmacol 2015;31(1):14–24.

Technology Basics for Telemedicine
What Practitioners Need to Know

Ashley Mitek, DVM, MS, DACVAA

KEYWORDS

- Medical technology • Telehealth • Telemedicine • Virtual veterinary care
- Artificial intelligence • Machine learning • Deep learning

KEY POINTS

- Telehealth technology is advancing at a rapid pace and shows great promise in helping veterinarians provide high-quality care.
- Artificial Intelligence will impact many aspects of veterinary medicine for the better.
- Approximately 4.9 billion people around the world (62% of the population) use the Internet. It is now possible for veterinarians to help patients anywhere with an Internet connection, making veterinary care more equitable and accessible.
- There are several challenges to overcome before the veterinary profession embraces new telemedicine technology. Education will be key to surpass our fears of technology.

INTRODUCTION

Technology is best when it brings people together.
—Matt Mullenweg, Creator of WordPress

The term veterinary medical technology relates to a range of tools that can enable the veterinary health care team to provide patients and society with a better quality of medicine. These tools may assist by contributing to early diagnosis, reducing complications, and optimizing treatment and overall, can facilitate the practice of veterinary medicine.[1] Because new technologies including high-speed Internet, video conferencing, and digital examination equipment have evolved, veterinary telemedicine (TM) is at the precipice of a revolution. This review focuses on the components of veterinary TM technology that primary care veterinarians should be familiar with.

In March 2020, the Centers for Medicare and Medicaid Services announced the need for providers to quickly pivot to TM in order to provide patients care in hospitals and other settings across the United States.[2] TM facilitates the intercommunication

Co-Founder, Stratocyte.com, Owner, AnesthesiaDiva.com, 48-113 Angel Wing Peak Glacier National Park, MT, USA
E-mail address: Diva@AnesthesiaDiva.com

Vet Clin Small Anim 52 (2022) 1109–1122
https://doi.org/10.1016/j.cvsm.2022.06.003
0195-5616/22/© 2022 Elsevier Inc. All rights reserved.
vetsmall.theclinics.com

between a health care provider and a patient, or, in the case of veterinary medicine, a veterinarian, pet owner, and a patient.

TM is often wrongly associated with futuristic or elaborate technological tools. Telemedicine is really the simple practice of caring for patients over distances. For as far back as 500 BCE, humans have been using messengers to transfer medical advice and pharmacueticals.[2] As technological advancements have developed, society has seen the benefit of the printing press, the telegraph, telephone, and the Internet. All have had a profound contribution to the advancement and accessibility of medical care. Human and veterinary patients alike can now receive live-chats in their home or use asynchronous ways to connect with health care professionals. Before the advent of smartphones, veterinarians may have thought of medical technology as an electrocardiogram or other tech device that is stand-alone, capturing specific patient data. But today, the field has exploded to include many more categories. Veterinary technology can more broadly be defined as the use of science to invent useful things or to solve problems.[3]

It is important to consider why TM developed when discussing the technology behind it. TM offers 5 advantages that are often termed the "5 C's": accessible care, increased convenience, enhanced comfort, greater confidentiality, and reduced risk of contagion.[4] The consumer's perceived advantages and needs will continually drive technology development further, in a positive feedback loop.

FACE YOUR FEARS FIRST

Knowledge is the antidote to fear.

—*Ralph Waldo Emerson*

Health care providers are often resistant to change. We are taught to practice evidence-based medicine, and sometimes, it takes time for that scientific evidence to be proved. Technology is rapidly evolving at a pace that is hard to keep up with. This speed often scares practitioners and is frequently coupled with a fear of being replaced. It's important to recognize how fear of technology can negatively affect a health care team before it is even rolled out.[5] Veterinarians are encouraged to face their fears of technology, in the spirit of continual professional growth and the quest to provide the best veterinary care possible. Technology will not replace veterinarians, but it does have the ability to make their job easier, if you befriend and understand it.

Administrators often drag their feet when it comes to making decisions about TM and making the leap to invest in such technology and strategies. Veterinary hospitals should attempt to practice the best quality medicine, and there is no doubt that in many situations, but not all, TM can be beneficial, facilitate the provision of high-quality care, and provide more accessible and equitable care to pets. Before jumping into TM, clinicians should identify their needs first and then search for vendors and software that fits the specific needs of their particular practice.

DEFINITIONS

Education is the best prescription for fear of the unknown. The following is an incomplete list of terms practitioners may want to be aware of, because they are either already using these technologies or will do so in the future. It is also likely that veterinarians will need to increasingly work with computer engineers and information technology experts to enhance the quality of care we can provide.

Medical technology: the application of science to develop solutions to health problems.[6] *Devices, procedures and systems are just a few of the ways medical technology
can solve health problems.*

Augmented veterinarian: clinicians who use their clinical experience as well as their
digital expertise to solve modern veterinary health problems. These individuals have
training not only in traditional veterinary medicine but also in computations sciences,
coding, algorithms, and mechatronic engineering[7]; this is the veterinarian of the future.

Broadband: a type of Internet connection that refers to wide bandwidth data transmission; this is a high-capacity transmission technique using a wide range of frequencies, which enables several messages to be communicated simultaneously;
this is the "passway" that data are moving on.[8]

Wi-Fi: Wi-Fi is not the same as Broadband. Wi-Fi can be understood as the means
by which broadband can be accessed wirelessly.[8] It's a group of wireless network
protocols, frequently used for local area networking of devices and Internet access.[9]
It uses radio frequencies and signals to transfer data without wires. In comparison,
broadband is the transmission of data with the use of high-speed Internet. All Wi-Fi
connections work on 2 frequency bands—2.4 Ghz and 5 Ghz.[8]

4G wireless data network: the fourth generation of broadband cellular network technology, succeeding 3G. 4G users experience speeds up to 100 Mbps.[10,11]

5G wireless data network: fifth generation technology standard for broadband
cellular networks. Cellular phone companies started deploying 5G in 2019. By 2025,
it is predicted that more than 1.7 subscribers worldwide will be connected using
5G.[12,13]

Fiber-Optic Internet: a broadband connection that can reach exceptional speeds,
with low lag time. It is a method of transmitting information using pulses of infrared
light through an optical fiber, which can send data as fast as 70% the speed of light.[14]

Satellite Internet: wireless internet from satellites orbiting Earth. Rural communities
and individuals in remote locations, who previously could not connect to the internet,
can now do so using satellites. One company, Starlink, is a satellite internet
constellation operated by SpaceX. They aim for global coverage sometime after 2023.

Artificial intelligence (AI): the ability of a digital computer or computer-controlled
robot to perform tasks commonly associated with intelligent beings.[15]

Machine Learning: a subfield of AI, which is broadly defined as the capability of a
machine to imitate intelligent human behavior.[16]

Deep learning: deep learning networks are neural networks with many layers. The
layered network can process extensive amounts of data and determine the "weight"
of each link in the network—for example, in an image recognition system (such as radiography), some layers of the neural network might detect individual features, whereas
another layer would be able to tell whether those features appear in a way that indicates a face. Deep learning is modeled on the way the human brain works and powers
many machine-learning uses, such as autonomous vehicles, chatbots, and medical
diagnostics.[17]

Natural language processing AI: natural language processing (NLP) is a branch of
computer science, and artifical intelligence, that gives computers the ability to understand text and spoken words in much the same way human beings can.[17]

Dehumanization of medicine: the denial of full humanness (identity and community) in
others and the cruelty and suffering that accompanies it.[18] Dehumanization frequently
ignores the patient's or client's individuality. Technology has the potential to dehumanize the practice of veterinary medicine.

Ambient clinical intelligence (ACI): physical spaces that are sensitive and responsive
to the presence of humans. The technology hinges on data collected by sensors and

processors embedded into everyday objects and uses machine learning algorithms for data analytics. For example, Google Assistant and Amazon Alexa are devices that automatically respond to a person's voice and use ambient intelligence.[19]

Carebot: robots designed to assist elderly people. An example is Honda's Asimo robot, which is an autonomous humanoid robot that can help patients by getting them food or turning off a light.[20] Carebots may be used in veterinary TM in the future.

Virtual Private Network (VPN): a way to connect to the internet over a public wireless connection that is secure and private.

Ambient Clinical Intelligence: ACI is a sensitive, adaptive, and responsive digital environment surrounding a doctor and the patient.[35] This technology makes it possible, for example, to analyze an interview with a client and automatically fill a patient's EMR.

TYPES OF VISITS

It is hard to talk about technology, as it relates to TM without briefly describing the types of TM available. Afterall, technology develops to solve a problem, and there are 3 types of TM categories that are commonly used in veterinary practice today. Each one of these has a specific use in practice and needs to be considered as you select the ideal platform(s) for your clinic. Undoubtedly, new strategies will develop to address consumer demand.

Remote Monitoring

Patient monitoring or population health management platforms identify biomedical measurements from patients. These data points are sent electronically to software algorithms that can then provide feedback to the pet owner or veterinary health care team.[21] These data can also be supervised by a veterinarian or veterinary health care professional.[22] Live video is rarely a component in these platforms. Patient data are often simple, and when a reading is outside of set parameters, an alert can be triggered, to the owner and/or veterinary team. RM can be helpful when discharging a postoperative patient from the hospital by recognizing and identifying changes in a patient's vital signs early. Home health aides, such as FitBit, Apple Health Kit, or Samsung Health should not be confused with RM, as they are not connected to a central monitoring system.[23]

Consultative Visits

Consultative visits are hallmarked by a conversation that does not necessarily require diagnostic tools to be used during the visit. A pet owner can confer directly with a veterinarian (direct-to-consumer or DTC), or a primary care veterinarian can confer directly with a specialist (teleconsultation or vet-to-specialist, VTS) in which the pet owner may or may not be present in a 3-way call. These conversations can be synchronous and occur via a live video or audio feed or can be asynchronous and occur in a chat box.

Specific types of consultative visits; these can be video, audio, or asynchronous (chat) based:

1. Client-to-vet (CTV): the pet owner and a member of the veterinary health care team communicate.
2. Vet-to-vet (VTV): the patient's primary care veterinarian confers directly with another veterinarian, such as a specialist, for a consultation on the case. Also known as a teleconsultation.

3. Vet-to-vet + client (VTV + C): similar to VTV, except the client is a participant in a 3-way video conference, audio call, or asynchronous chat, with both the primary care veterinarian and the other veterinarian, who may be a specialist consulting on the case.

Consultative visits have several benefits, including facilitating communication between all parties who could be located geographically in different areas and time zones. A secure and reliable connection is mandatory for consultative visits.

Direct to Consumer

Direct to consumer (DTC) is a rapidly evolving segment of the industry and represents a variation of a CTV type of consultative visit. But it deserves a unique mention because these companies offer apps that allow a pet owner to directly connect with a veterinarian who they may have never seen before and do not have an established veterinarian-client-patient relationship. Most of these apps use interactive video or chat between a patient and an on-demand veterinarian. Clients typically use a smartphone or laptop to connect. Fees are typically paid upfront for the visit, and the client will wait in an online queue before information exchanges between the parties. Most diagnostic tools are not available for most DTC platforms, and veterinarians are limited by the information supplied by the pet owner. Urgent care and triage cases use DTC platforms most frequently.

DTC can be particularly helpful to veterinary practices that do not have the staff to offer after hours emergency services or triage care. In that situation, the practice can outsource these cases to a DTC operation. Veterinarian workflows are typically set rigidly in these DTC platforms, and they are limited to triage situations.

FACILITATED VIRTUAL VISITS ARE COMING

A physical examination can be performed remotely with the appropriate hardware, software, and staffing. With a facilitated virtual visit, cameras, electronic stethoscopes, and robots or human support staff/facilitator can palpate and procure images and sounds for a remote veterinarian to evaluate. These platforms use something called Provider Access Software.[3] In human medicine, this software allows for the integration of Class 1 and sometimes Class 2 medical devices into live streams. A Class 1 device is one that has low-to-moderate risk for patient use. And a Class 2 device is a device that has moderate-to-high risk for patient use. Digital stethoscopes, telemetry, wireless blood pressure devices, and otoscopes are examples of medical devices that could be integrated into a facilitated virtual visit.

Another option is for a technician or other animal health care team member to physically go to the patient's home (also known as the "originating site") to collect the needed information and relay that information back to the veterinarian using the platform. These individuals are typically referred to as "facilitators" for the purposes of virtual visits. The facilitator can serve as the extension of a clinician doing the examination and ensure the medical devices are used appropriately. For example, a technician is sent to do a physical examination, collect vital signs and bloodwork, and that information is relayed to the veterinarian. Facilitators can be technicians or other individuals who have been trained by the veterinary health care team.

Facilitated virtual visits may make veterinary care more accessible to pets who otherwise cannot travel, may facilitate the more frequent evaluation of a pet, and reduce hospital readmissions and identify abnormal conditions sooner. Patients in rural settings that are underserved can particularly benefit from these visits. In human medicine, facilitated virtual visits are particularly helpful in jails and prisons, as well as schools and workplaces.[23] These captive or semicaptive settings are often ideal as remote TM clinics that are staffed with a facilitator and no doctor. Doggie day care, grooming, and boarding facilities are examples of semicaptive environments that may lend themselves well to this workflow.

TECHNICAL AND SUPPORT STAFF ARE ESSENTIAL

The technical aspects of starting a TM program are daunting. The most common cause for a failed leap into the TM world is often due to frustrations arising from the lack of support when technical difficulties arise. In addition to staff receiving training on how to best integrate TM into their practice and workflow, technical support staff must be available to immediately troubleshoot problems that arise; this can be handled one of two ways. First, the vendor you choose to use often offers technical support staff. Second, if your vendor does not offer this option, practices can hire a technical support staff member to manage technological transformation within their practice or outsource that to a remote virtual care support firm.

These IT individuals should be knowledgeable of video conferencing platforms, and it is often helpful for them to have some veterinary medical background, although on-the-job experience can be gained quite rapidly in a busy hospital. Veterinary technicians who have an interest or a background in technology are often ideal in these settings. The author is aware of several hospitals that have used this approach to "grow their own" internal staff member(s) devoted to medical technology troubleshooting; this can be a full- or part-time position.

Having a technical support person should not be considered a luxury in a veterinary hospital. It is a necessity today. It is also helpful if these IT hires possess great communication skills and are comfortable interacting within the walls of busy and dynamic veterinary hospitals. Their skill set should include the basics of understanding how video works, networking, firewalls, and basic computer skills.[23]

Adapting to new technology is often very frustrating and hard. But those hurdles can be overcome with appropriate training, patience and support personnel.

INTEGRATION INTO THE ELECTRONIC MEDICAL RECORD

Perhaps one of the greatest challenges facing veterinary medicine is the diversity of electronic medical record systems. Many practices have transitioned to electronic medical records (EMRs); however, a significant percentage of hospitals still use antiquated software, or paper records, or a combination of the both. In the ideal situation, a TM platform would seamlessly integrate into the hospital's medical record system.

In addition, it would be ideal if patient data (from wearable devices, patient records, and diagnostics, etc...) could all seamlessly integrate into one EMR that jives with TM, and then all of that data is stored in the cloud. This option does not yet exist in veterinary medicine but is likely to be available in the future as the technology adopts to consumer demand.

OPEN AND CLOSED SYSTEMS

One of the decisions that should be made when choosing between TM providers is picking between an open or closed system. An open system is one that allows the user to integrate various components of hardware and software from multiple different third-party sources. A closed system is one that all components, both the hardware and software, are designed, developed, and provided by one single manufacturer. Closed systems do not rely on third party sources.[7]

Administrators should weigh the pros and cons of both systems. Closed systems can often be more specialized, with streamlined workflows that are specific to a certain area of practice. Closed systems may be more "simple" and user friendly because they were created by one manufacturer. However, on the flip side, they often are inflexible and are less adaptable.

Open systems allow you to integrate different devices and softwares into the mix to customize a TM program for your practice. Users can develop their own workflows. Integration of new medical devices is also a pro of open systems. Because technology develops and becomes accessible to pet owners and veterinarians alike (such as wearable devices), it is more likely that these third-party systems could be integrated into an open system.

SATELLITE TELEMEDICINE CLINICS

Most veterinarians are familiar with the traditional model of veterinary care. A pet owner brings their animal into a clinic. At the other extreme of this is TM, where a pet owner may do a video conference call or asynchronous chat with the veterinarian. But this is far too black and white of a dynamic for what is the limitless bounds of using telehealth.

Practitioners who service rural areas or have an interest in servicing certain geographic regions can open satellite TM sites. A veterinarian does not need to be at this location, but instead, a trained veterinary support person (a TM "facilitator") is. At this location, the facilitator can attach the necessary devices and ensure appropriate video and audio connectivity for the practitioner to do a remote physical examination, communicate with the client, and direct any urgent interventions as needed. These facilitators can be trained to acquire diagnostic images and implement treatments, while being remotely supervised by a licensed veterinarian.

VIRTUAL PHYSICAL EXAMINATION

When TM initially entered the human medical and veterinary medical fields, many practitioners opined that a physical examination could never be completed without physically being present with the patient and the pet owner. Technology has proved this logic completely false. In fact, it is possible to do a complete physical examination remotely.

Table 1 describes the vital signs and physical examination parameters that can be assessed and evaluated remotely with the aid of a facilitator and/or the client's assistance.

RAPIDITY OF TECHNOLOGICAL ADVANCEMENTS

TM is advancing at an incredibly rapid pace. As Internet connectivity becomes faster and more accessible, it provides profound increases in the availability of veterinarians to help more people and animals, especially those that are underserved.

All TM technologies require an Internet connection. For many years, this was a severely limiting step in providing virtual health care to people and pets around the world. However, practitioners can now take their own internet connection with them wherever they go. 4G LTE and 5G wireless data networks operated by the various carriers provide outstanding coverage in many locations. And remote areas can now use satellite internet, making TM accessible nearly anywhere in the world. Veterinarians can have secure access to the EMR, do live TM sessions, and make an IP office desk phone work wherever they are.[23]

Table 1
Physical Examination

Categories	In-Person Technique	Virtual Technique @ Satellite Clinic
Mentation	Observe patient in the examination room	Same
Ophthalmic	Observe eyes	Facilitator uses an HD camera for veterinarian
Ears/Otoscopic/Dermatologic	Visual observation ± otoscopic examination	Facilitator uses an HD camera for Veterinarian ± digital otoscopic images
Lymph node palpation	Palpation by veterinarian	Facilitator is trained to identify LNs and measure sizes
Thoracic auscultation	Auscultation with stethoscope	Facilitator holds digital stethoscope to thorax
Thyroid	Palpation	Facilitator is trained to palpate and measure
Cardiac auscultation	Auscultation with stethoscope	Facilitator is trained to place digital stethoscope
Oral/MM/CRT	Visual observation	HD camera/visual observation with facilitator/owner assistance
Abdominal palpation	Palpation by veterinarian	Facilitator can be trained to assess for abdominal pain ± acquire flash ultrasound images
Vital signs (temperature, pulse, respiration)	Palpation/visual observation	Visual observation/palpation with facilitator assistance

Additional Diagnostics for Potential Urgent Care/Triage

	In-Person Technique	Virtual Technique @ Satellite Clinic
Pulse oximetry	Staff places and reads	Staff places and sends data to veterinarian
EKG	Staff places and reads	Staff places and sends data to veterinarian
Blood pressure	Staff places and reads	Staff places and sends data to veterinarian
Bloodwork	Staff collects and runs	Staff collects and runs, sends data to veterinarian for interpretation
Flash ultrasound	Veterinarian performs and interprets	Staff can perform and veterinarian can interpret images via video conference

Many major cities are becoming fiber connected and provide Internet speeds that are incredibly fast and reliable. One Gigabit per second is often easily available and is significantly faster than what is needed for TM. Some experts believe that 3D video may eventually replace the HD video conferencing currently available in most TM systems.[23]

ARTIFICIAL INTELLIGENCE

AI is the ability of a computer or a robot controlled by a computer to do tasks that are usually done by humans because they require human intelligence and discernment.[11] AI-powered medical technology is rapidly evolving into many solutions for clinical practice.[14] Certain specific conditions in clinical practice benefit currently from AI, but we will see those horizons exponentially expand in coming years. The detection of atrial fibrillation, epilepsy, seizures, and hypoglycemia are some of the areas where AI is beneficial. In addition, AI is available for medical imaging and histopathological examination too.

There are 3 types of AI[12,24]:

1. Artificial narrow intelligence (ANI or "weak AI") is focused on performing a specific task, and any information gained from that task will not be applied to other tasks (eg. Siri, Alexa, Facial recognition software, etc...). It is the only type of artificial intelligence we have successfully realized to date.
2. Artificial general intelligence (AGI or "strong AI"): is the hypothetical concept of a machine with general intelligence that mimics human intelligence and/or behaviours, with the ability to learn and apply its intelligence to solve any problem. To date, strong AI has not been achievable.
3. Artificial Super Intelligence (ASI): is hypothetical AI that doesn't just mimic or understand human intelligence and behaviour; it's when machines become self-aware and surpass the capacity of any human's intelligence and ability.

Machine learning and deep learning are two terms that are often used when discussing artificial intelligence, but they are not synonymous. An oversimplified yet concise definition is, machine learning is AI that can automatically adapt with minimal human interference. Deep learning is a subset of machine learning that uses artificial neural networks to mimic the learning process of the human brain

Deep learning and machine learning are subfields of artificial intelligence that have implications on the future of veterinary medicine and telehealth (**Figs 1** and **2**). Therefore, they deserve a brief description. Machine learning is a subfield of artificial intelligence that uses sample data, and learns from that data, then applies that new knowledge to make a decsion (email filters or speech recognition are examples of this). Deep learning is a subfield of machine learning. "Deep" refers to a neural network that has more than 3 layers. A "neural network" is simply a mimicry of the way a brain makes a decision, with a similar structure to how biological neurons signal to each other. Deep learning (such as self driving cars) can learn and make smart decisions on its own, but machine learning needs a human's help to process data.[1]

Advantages of AI[24]

- Reduce human error
- Available 24/7
- Assists with repetitive work
- Faster decision-making
- Rational decisions
- Communicates efficiently

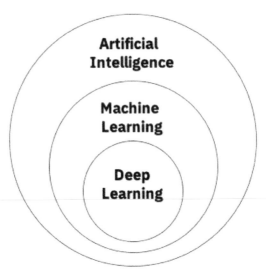

Fig. 1. Deep learning and machine learning are subfields of AI. (*From* Artificial Intelligence (AI), by IBM Cloud Education. June 3, 2020. https://www.ibm.com/cloud/learn/what-is-artificial-intelligence. Reprint Courtesy of IBM Corporation © 2020.).

We will continue to see the impact of AI on veterinary medicine. Everything from TM, to robot-assisted surgery, and vitals monitoring will likely be affected.[24] AI-powered technology is often said to enable the 4P model of medicine: Predictive, Preventative, Personalized, and Participatory.[25]

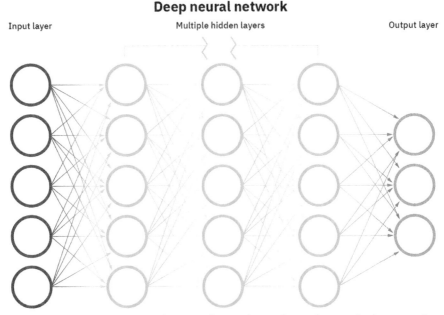

Fig. 2. Deep learning is a particular type of AI made up of neural networks that are at least 3 layers deep (*From* Artificial Intelligence (AI), by IBM Cloud Education. June 3, 2020. https://www.ibm.com/cloud/learn/what-is-artificial-intelligence. Reprint Courtesy of IBM Corporation © 2020.).

AI will certainly play a significant role in veterinary medicine in the near future. However, health care professionals are notoriously resistant to such technology,[26] and it is likely the field of veterinary medicine will likely experience the same cultural challenges. This phenomenon of physicians failing to accept new AI technology despite proven benefits is often explained by 4 causes. First, most veterinarians lack continuing education and training in this field.[7] Second, early digitization of health care flows came with a significant increase in administrative burden, which leads to increased veterinarian burnout.[27,28] Third, there is increasing fear as to the risk of AI replacing veterinarians entirely (realistically, AI will complement a veterinarian's intelligence, not replace it[29–31]). Lastly, there is a lack of legal framework that defines the concept of liability in the case of adoption or rejection of algorithm recommendations.[32]

It is clear that veterinary schools will need to adapt to these challenges and educate future veterinarians about AI. Several medical schools have started to incorporate engineering and AI into the medical curriculum.[33,34]

THE DEHUMANIZATION OF VETERINARY MEDICINE

AI does not dehumanize humans — humans do.

—Xianto Wang

As technology progresses, it is natural for our profession to stop and address the topic of dehumanization, which anecdotally is a fear reported by veterinarians.

Will veterinarians be replaced by AI? No. It is likely, however, that the traditional model of veterinary care will be augmented by AI, and the veterinarian will be assisted by smart medical technologies. AI outperforms humans, but only in low-level tasks.[36] Veterinarians are encouraged to look at AI as an additional tool in their tool kit, just as digital radiography, or virtual teleconsultations with a specialist, can allow them to practice high-quality medicine in a more efficient manner. Additional research is needed on this topic to help the veterinary profession better understand how to adapt to and best use AI.

The dehumanization of veterinary medicine is often perceived as a threat and a bad thing. But dehumanization of care can have benefits; this is particularly true if you have to interview owners about questions that could induce shame or other negative emotions they are embarrassed by.[37,38] Humans also make errors, and AI technologies are less likely to be affected by the subjectivity of the human mind. Nevertheless, the profession will need to remain vigilant about dehumanization as technology develops.

SUMMARY

Technology is nothing. What's important is that you have faith in people, that they're basically good and smart, and if you give them tools, they'll do wonderful things with them.

—Steve Jobs

Telemedicine technology has the ability to enhance the way veterinary medicine is practiced and progress the field in leaps and bounds. The increasing availability of high-speed Internet will continue to make veterinary care more accessible, and specific TM software and hardware will be innovated to meet these opportunities for growth. Veterinarians will increasingly use AI to practice their craft in a more efficient manner. Strap on your seatbelt folks — veterinary medicine is being thrust into a new age of tech!

CLINICS CARE POINTS

- Advancing telehealth technology allows for more accesible veterinary care and increased convenience to pet owners.
- Change is hard. When adopting new telehealth initiatives or deploying new technology in your practice, be patient.
- Advancing telemedicine technology and artificial intelligence will continue to impact veterinary medicine. Increased accessibility of care and data transmission will increase the demand for veterinarians and healthcare providers in the future.

DISCLOSURES

A. Mitek is a co-founder of Stratocyte.com, a virtual marketplace that connects veterinary specialists with primary care veterinarians around the world. She also owns AnesthesiaDiva.com and provides anesthesia teleconsultations and training to veterinary healthcare providers globally.

REFERENCES

1. IBM Cloud Education. Artificial Intelligence. 2020. Available at: https://www.ibm.com/cloud/learn/what-is-artificial-intelligence. Accessed December 20, 2021.
2. Jin MX, Kim SY, Miller LJ, et al. Telemedicine: current impact on the future. Cureus 2020;12(8):e9891.
3. Merriam-Webster. Available at: https://www.merriam-webster.com/dictionary/technology. Accessed December 20, 2021.
4. Dorsey ER, Okun MS, Bloem BR. Care, convenience, comfort, confidentiality, and contagion: the 5 C's that will shape the future of telemedicine. J Parkinsons Dis 2020;10:893–7.
5. Baker J, Anthony S. Telemedicine technology: a review of services, equipment, and other aspects. Curr Allergy Asthma Rep 2018;11:1–8.
6. Tulchinsky TH, Varavikova EA. Health technology, quality, law, and ethics. The New Public Health 2014;771–819. https://doi.org/10.1016/B978-0-12-415766-8.00015-X.
7. Haag M, Igel C, Fischer MR. German Medical Education Society (GMA) "Digitization-Technology-Assisted Learning and Teaching" joint working group "Technology-enhanced Teaching and Learning in Medicine (TeLL)" of the german association for medical informatics biometry and epidemiology (gmds) and the German Informatics Society (GI). Digital teaching and digital medicine: a national initiative is needed. GMS J Med Educ 2018;35:Doc43.
8. Broadband vs Wifi: What's the difference. 2020. Available at: https://www.actcorp.in/blog/difference-between-wifi-and-broadband. Accessed December 20, 2021.
9. Wi-Fi. Wikipedia. Available at: https://en.wikipedia.org/wiki/Wi-Fi. Accessed December 20, 2021.
10. What is SD-WAN, and what does it mean for networking, security, cloud?. Available at: https://www.networkworld.com/article/3031279/sd-wan-what-it-is-and-why-you-ll-use-it-one-day.html. Accessed December 20, 2021.
11. 4G Wikipedia. 2022. Available at: https://en.wikipedia.org/wiki/4G. Accessed December 20, 2021.

12. 5 G Wikipedia. 2022. Available at: https://en.wikipedia.org/wiki/5G. Accessed December 20, 2021.
13. "Positive 5G Outlook Post COVID-19: What Does It Mean for Avid Gamers?". Forest Interactive. November 13, 2020. Accessed December 21, 2022. https://www.forest-interactive.com/newsroom/positive-5g-outlook-post-covid-19-what-does-it-mean-for-avid-gamers/
14. Understanding Wavelengths In Fiber Optics. Available at: https://www.centurylink.com/home/help/internet/fiber/what-is-fiber-internet.html. Accessed December 16, 2019.
15. Artificial Intelligence. Encyclopedia Britannica. Available at: https://www.britannica.com/technology/artificial-intelligence. Accessed December 20, 2021.
16. Brown, Sara. Machine Learning Explained. 2021. Available at: https://mitsloan.mit.edu/ideas-made-to-matter/machine-learning-explained. Accessed December 20, 2021.
17. What is Natural Language. IBM. 2020. Available at: https://www.ibm.com/cloud/learn/natural-language-processing. Accessed December 20, 2021.
18. Haslam N. Dehumanization: An Integrative Review. Personal Social Psychol Rev 2006;10(3):252–64. Archived from the original on 2020-09-10. Retrieved 2019-06-22 – via Lawrence Erlbaum Associates, Inc, Accessed December 20, 2021.
19. Available at: https://ehrintelligence.com/features/ambient-clinical-intelligence-what-it-means-for-the-ehr-industry. Accessed December 20, 2021.
20. Available at: https://www.businessinsider.com/japan-developing-carebots-for-elderly-care-2015-11. Accessed December 20, 2021.
21. Barrett M, Combs V, Su JG, et al. AIR Louisville: addressing asthma with technology, crowdsourcing, cross-sector collaboration, and policy. Health Aff (Millwood) 2018;37(4):525–34. Available at: https://doi-org.proxy2.library.illinois.edu/10.1377/hlthaff.2017.1315.
22. Kim MY, Lee SY, Jo EJ, et al. Feasibility of a smartphone application based action plan and monitoring in asthma. Asia Pac Allergy 2016;6(3):174–80. Available at: https://doi-org.proxy2.library.illinois.edu/10.5415/apallergy.2016.6.3.174.
23. Baker. Available at. https://link-springer-com.proxy2.library.illinois.edu/article/10.1007/s11882-018-0814-6. Accessed December 20, 2021.
24. What is Artificial Intelligence? How does AI work, Types and Future of it?. 2021. Available at: https://www.mygreatlearning.com/blog/what-is-artificial-intelligence/. Accessed December 20, 2021.
25. Orth M, Averina M, Chatzipanagiotou S, et al. Opinion: redefining the role of the physician in laboratory medicine in the context of emerging technologies, personalised medicine and patient autonomy ('4P medicine'). J Clin Pathol 2019;72:191–7.
26. Briganti G, Le Moine O. Artificial intelligence in medicine: today and tomorrow. Front Med 2020;7. Available at: https://www.frontiersin.org/articles/10.3389/fmed.2020.00027/full.
27. Chaiyachati KH, Shea JA, Asch DA, et al. Assessment of inpatient time allocation among first-year internal medicine residents using time-motion observations. JAMA Int Med 2019;179:760–7.
28. West CP, Dyrbye LN, Shanafelt TD. Physician burnout: contributors, consequences and solutions. J Intern Med 2018;283:516–29.
29. Shah NR. Health care in 2030: will artificial intelligence replace physicians? Ann Intern Med 2019;170:407–8.

30. Topol EJ. High-performance medicine: the convergence of human and artificial intelligence. Nat Med 2019;25:44–56.
31. Verghese A, Shah NH, Harrington RA. What this computer needs is a physician: humanism and artificial intelligence. JAMA 2018;319:19–20.
32. Price WN, Gerke S, Cohen IG. Potential liability for physicians using artificial intelligence. JAMA 2019;322:1765–6.
33. Briganti G. Nous Devons Former des Médecins ≪ augmentés ≫. France (Paris): Le Specialiste.; 2019. Available at. https://www.lespecialiste.be/fr/debats/nous-devons-former-des-medecins-laquo-nbsp-augmentes-raquo.html.   Accessed October 26, 2019.
34. Brouillette M. AI added to the curriculum for doctors-to-be. Nat Med 2019;25:1808–9.
35. Acampora G, Cook DJ, Rashidi P, et al. A survey on ambient intelligence in health care. Proc IEEE Inst Elect Electron Eng 2013;101:2470–94.
36. Wang X. Artificial Intelligence and the Loss of Humanity. 2020. Available at: https://bpr.berkeley.edu/2020/11/15/artificial-intelligence-and-the-loss-of-humanity/. Accessed December 20, 2021.
37. Palmer A, Schwan D. Beneficent dehumanization: Employing artificial intelligence and carebots to mitigate shame-induced barriers to medical care. Bioethics 2022;36(2):187–93. Epub 2021 Dec 23. PMID: 34942057.
38. Tuckson RV, Edmunds M, Hodgkins ML. Telehealth. N Engl J Med 2017;377(16):1585–92.

Telehealth in Hospice and Palliative Care

Shea Cox, DVM, CVPP, CHPV, RN*

KEYWORDS

- Telehospice • Telepalliative care • Palliative care • Hospice • Veterinary
- Telehealth

KEY POINTS

- Telehealth-based interventions can improve the remote delivery of hospice and palliative care to patients.
- Clients oftentimes wish for their pet to receive hospice and palliative care in the home setting, and telehealth can be used to support this goal.
- A virtual care platform can significantly increase the level of communication and contact between the client and hospice and palliative care providers, increasing feelings of connectedness, security, and trust.
- Evidence-based palliative care communication strategies can be used for more effective communication when using telehealth modalities, including building rapport and establishing trust with clients navigating serious illness in their pet.

INTRODUCTION

Hospice and palliative care is medical care focused on the palliation of a patient's pain and symptoms while attending to the emotional and spiritual needs of the client caregiver.

Hospice is a specific type of palliative care for terminal patients who likely have six or fewer months to live and where clients no longer wish to pursue curative treatments.

Palliative care, on the other hand, can be provided at any stage of illness, regardless of prognosis, or whether a patient continues to receive curative care or treatment aimed at slowing the progression of disease. Not all palliative care is hospice, although hospice care is always palliative.

Hospice and palliative care is best delivered in-home by an interdisciplinary team (IDT). In veterinary medicine, the IDT ideally consists of a veterinarian, veterinary nurse, care coordinator, and social worker at minimum. The key roles of the IDT include supporting effective pain and symptom management in the veterinary patient, identifying

BluePearl Pet Hospice, Blue Pearl Specialty and Emergency Pet Hospital, 2950 Busch Lake Boulevard, Tampa, FL 33614, USA
* Corresponding author.
E-mail address: shea.cox@bluepearlvet.com

Vet Clin Small Anim 52 (2022) 1123–1133
https://doi.org/10.1016/j.cvsm.2022.05.002
0195-5616/22/© 2022 Elsevier Inc. All rights reserved.

and addressing clients' goals of care, providing access to psychosocial support and bereavement care for family members, and supporting other veterinary care providers who are also involved in patient and client care.

Telehealth is a critical service addition for the delivery of high-quality, home-based hospice and palliative care. When used for patients at end of life, telehealth improves access to care and allows for more timely clinical interventions, which in turn improves patient quality of life through better clinical management. It empowers clients the ability to manage their pet's illness which decreases the need for in-hospital visits, allowing compromised patients to remain at home while still receiving the care needed.

Telehospice and telepalliative care, specifically, are the application of telehealth technologies to hospice and palliative care and can take many forms including video-conferencing, telephonic communication, or remote symptom monitoring, and it can address the many needs of both patients and clients.

DISCUSSION
Clinical Relevance

The diagnosis of a life-limiting illness, along with its management during periods of wellness, illness, remission, and decline can be stressful for both clients and the veterinary health care teams. Utilization of telehealth technology at a patient's end of life can help.

The utilization of telehealth to deliver hospice and palliative care improves client access to the IDT, contributing to feelings of connectedness, security, and trust toward their veterinary care providers, which is critical for the patient and vital for client satisfaction.

Telehealth also extends clinical reach by providing care when and where it is needed regardless of location; limits patient and caregiver travel time, expense, and time away from work; improves outcomes through timely care and immediate access to the care team; relieves caregiver burden; and promotes greater patient, client, and provider satisfaction.

Telehealth can help build connections between the veterinary team and client, mitigate uncertainty in care, help assess and manage symptoms in a timely manner, determine care priorities in the face of life-threatening illness, and promote comfort, connectedness, and dignity during a pet's last phase of life.

How Telehealth Can Support the Delivery of Hospice and Palliative Care

Telehospice and telepalliative care improves patient care access, reduces client illness-related burden, offers real-time monitoring and management of symptoms, and proactively identify clinical decline. Although technology does not completely replace in-person encounters, it can offer meaningful connection and bridge gaps in patient and client care in the following ways:

- Telehealth extends clinical reach by providing care when and where it is needed, improving clinical outcomes through timely care and immediate access to the care team.
- Telehealth supplements in-person visits and provides an important way to connect with patients and clients, especially those who live far away or have pets that are too debilitated to attend an in-clinic appointment.
- Telehealth improves communication between clients and the IDT, which improves pain and symptom management and increases client satisfaction.[1]
- Telehealth-based interventions have been associated with improved clinical outcomes through improving client compliance rates.[2]

- Telehealth allows for education and coaching of client caregivers when it is needed and opportunity for goals of care discussions and emotional support.
- Telehealth can be used to support other veterinary care providers who are with a patient in the home, such as a veterinary nurse performing an in-home assessment under the veterinarian's guidance.
- Telehealth helps address challenges in veterinary medicine such as staffing shortages, work–life balance, burnout, and compassion fatigue.

Clinical Applications of Telehospice and Telepalliative Care

In hospice and palliative care, every patient is different and has unique needs, with some patient and clients' needs being greater and more frequent than others. The utilization of telehealth allows the IDT to communicate better with clients who may need attention more often than an in-person veterinary team member can provide. Telehealth provides real-time support to the patient and client and expands the reach of the veterinary provider, enhancing communication and the patient–client experience.

Improved access can lead to improved quality of care and less acute care needs which are often present in the hospice or palliative care patient. It can also provide continuity of care and address urgent concerns, which is a common occurrence as a patient nears the end of life.

Listed are a few examples of how telehospice and telepalliative care can be used for the care of an end-of-life patient and client:

- *Patients with chronic conditions or comorbidities:* Telehealth can supplement in-person visits to provide continuity of care and it allows the veterinary team to address urgent concerns which are common as a patient nears the end of life.
- *Symptom management:* Telehealth allows for a real-time assessment of patients from an environment where they are most comfortable and where clinical symptoms are not as readily masked. Because clinical interventions can sometimes be as simple as a medication change, telehealth allows near instant treatment and relief of symptoms for the comfort of the pet and for the convenience of the client (**Fig. 1**).
- *Environmental modifications to support comfort and quality of life:* Telehealth allows the veterinary team to continually observe the patient in its home environment and assess social interactions between other pets and people in the home which can provide broader insights impacting end-of-life care.
- *Client education:* The level of client caregiver anxiety can be alleviated when proper education is provided. Telehealth lends itself nicely to client education through virtual observation and can help guide them in real-time, providing an additional layer of support during a challenging time. An example would be providing education and guidance as a client is performing subcutaneous fluid administration or giving injections.
- *Client support:* Telehealth allows the opportunity for continued conversations around advanced care planning including goals of care, euthanasia planning, and decision-making. It is critical to frequently revisit these conversations, which do not need to take place in an in-clinic setting.

A 10-Step Framework for Successful Telehospice or Telepalliative Care Visits

Hospice and palliative care consultations have important nuances that differ from other types of clinical encounters. The following 10-step framework will provide basic guidelines to help ensure a successful virtual visit.

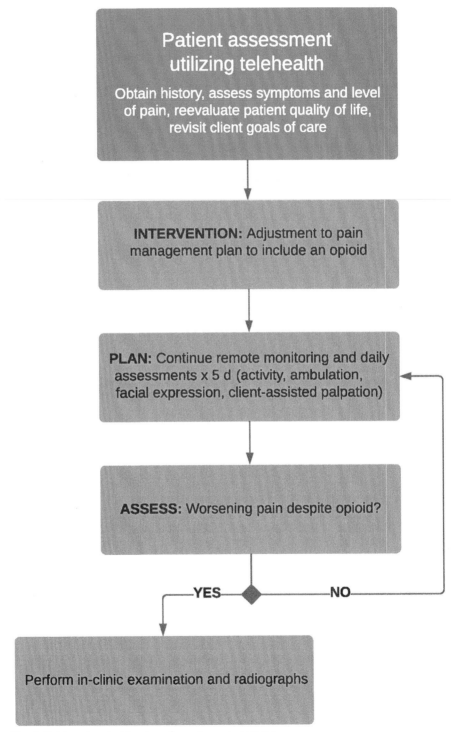

Fig. 1. Telehospice decision tree for pain management.

Step 1: Prepare
- If possible, hospice and palliative care virtual visits should be via video and not a phone call. Video-based delivery of telehealth is associated with stronger relationships and shared trust between clients and providers compared with audio-only delivery, which is critical for hospice and palliative care relationships.[3]
- Identify a team member, such as a veterinary nurse or assistant, to prepare and educate the client before the appointment to ensure the visit runs smoothly. This is especially important if you are connecting with a client for the first time. Preparation should include sharing information about the length and goals of the visit, making sure that technology is working for the client, and providing the client with a backup plan if there is a technology fail, such as using a phone call to connect.
- For navigating delicate end-of-life conversations, it is crucial to be able to appreciate body language and subtle facial expressions. Because of this, avoid using small devices, such as smartphones or tablets, which can limit your visual assessments. Instead, use a laptop or desktop computer with a high-quality webcam and microphone and maximize the client on your computer screen to give the best chance of interpreting nonverbal cues.
- Make sure you are against a warm, neutral background, and wear clothing that is free of patterns which can be distracting on video.
- Providers and clients should avoid backlighting as this darkens faces, making it difficult to see and interpret expressions.

Step 2: Personalize
- In hospice situations, it is important to personalize introductions to establish connection and rapport. Introduce yourself by name and acknowledge the use of technology during a sensitive and intimate time. Assure your client that you are present and "with them" despite not being in the same room. Phrases such as, "*I may not be with you in person, but I'm here to support you across the distance*" can be powerful for clients to hear and help set them at ease.
- Spend the first 3-to-5 minutes of your visit sharing something personal about yourself to establish connection: "*I understand you live in Berkeley; my husband and I recently moved from there and now live in Temecula. I do miss the area; what is it that you like best about it?*"

Step 3: Frame
- It is important to begin a consult by sharing a timeframe and asking what the client wishes to discuss: "*We will have an hour together and I wanted to begin by asking you what your goals are for today's visit. What concerns you would like to be sure that we explore in-depth together?*" This approach helps set expectations, frames the conversation, ensures that you are taking into consideration clients' needs, and sets a tone of client-centered care, which is important in hospice and palliative care situations.
- If you as the provider have specific topics you need to include, ask permission. "*Thank you for sharing what is most important for you today, we will be sure to cover that. In addition to those things, I would also like to discuss my concerns that Max may be experiencing some discomfort. Would that be OK?*"

Step 4: Understand
- It is important to explore where your clients have been and what they currently understand.
- Ask what other veterinary care providers have been involved in care, including specialists and/or any emergency visits.

- Find out what they understand about their pet's medical condition and what has been offered thus far. Use open-ended questions such as, "*Share with me what you understand about Max's diagnosis of bone cancer, his osteosarcoma. What options have been discussed with you?*" Avoid closed-ended questions such as, "*Do you understand the diagnosis of Max's bone cancer?*" Vital information can be missed when a client responds with a "yes" or "no" answer.
- If you need to review the medical record and/or document during the visit, ask permission to divert your attention. Use phrases such as, "*What you just shared with me is important and I want to make sure I capture it. Please excuse me while I type this information. I'm still here with you.*" If you do not communicate this, you risk looking distracted or not fully present, which can erode the trust and connection critical to end-of-life relationships.

Step 5: Assess

- In addition to client communications, goals for the hospice and palliative care consult are to assess both the pet and the environment in which they live.
- Virtually examine the patient by guiding clients to move their device as needed, instructing them how to touch, press, or show their pet according to your instructions.
- Ask permission to scan the environment. Ask clients to "walk" you around their home to areas where their pet sleeps, eats, eliminates, or any other important areas such as stairs or yard.

Step 6: Verify

- It is important to review and verify current medications for accuracy. Ask clients to show you all the medications their pet is taking, including OTC and supplements, to ensure accuracy with what is documented in the pet's medical record.
- Polypharmacy is common in hospice and palliative care patients. Take this time to explore if there are any challenges with medication delivery, such as refusal of medications or difficulty administering certain forms of medications, an incompatible schedule with regard to medication administration times or frequency, or caregiver overwhelm with the number of medications prescribed.

Step 7: Signpost

- Ending a telehealth visit can believe abrupt or awkward and because of this, it is especially important in hospice situations to use a communication signpost such as, "*We have about 10 minutes left together. What might be most helpful for you to discuss before we end our conversation for today?*" This helps mentally prepare the client for the end of the visit and return focus to the specific needs of the client.

Step 8: Summarize

- Clients often believe a sense of "mental overwhelm" during emotionally difficult end-of-life conversations, and adding to this is the fact that most people's attention spans are generally short. Because of this, it is imperative to summarize and review what was covered: "*During our time together we discussed that your number one goal for Max was comfort, and because of that, we are going to adjust his pain management plan beginning this evening.*"
- Verbalize the follow-up actions you will take before ending the visit. "*I will be dispensing a new medication for Max today to better control his discomfort. I will update your veterinarian and oncologist with the changes to his care plan. You will be receiving a copy of this plan within the next 24 hours but don't hesitate to reach out if you have any questions or concerns prior to this time.*"
- To ensure understanding, ask clients to repeat back to you what was shared.
- Share your written care plan and next steps in a digital format with the client. Clients should ideally receive a written summary within 24 hours of the virtual visit.

Step 9: Plan
- Be sure to plan follow-up visits. Client communication and education are improved with more frequent, brief encounters. In hospice and palliative care situations, 20- to 30-min weekly check-ins are recommended which can be performed by the veterinary nurse following the initial consultation.
- Ensure that there is a protocol in place for any issues that may arise.

Step 10: Document
- Document your medical record for a telehealth visit just as you would any in-person visit, according to your Veterinary State Practice Act.
- With regard to telehealth-specific documentation, ensure to note the type of visit performed (video, telephone, asynchronous vs synchronous) and indicate that the patient's needs are being met with the use of telehealth.

Hospice and Palliative Care Communication Tips when Using Telehealth

Telehealth technology is an essential tool for the delivery of veterinary hospice and palliative care; however, a question as to whether telehealth can think too detached to be useful in the intimate world of end-of-life care is a fair one to be raised. In answer to that question, studies in human medicine have shown that virtual visits do not compromise the quality of hospice and palliative care being delivered, and that virtual visits are as effective as in-person visits.[4] It can be reasonably extrapolated that a similar experience is had by clients engaging in hospice and palliative care services for their pet, and when paired with quality in-home and/or in-clinic care, telehealth can further enhance the "personal" experience that is so often associated with hospice and palliative medicine.

With regard to "humanizing technology" for more compassionate communications, there are many ways the veterinary team can adopt effective techniques during video visits to compensate for the lack of physical presence. Although many communication skills are universal, some must be adapted to accommodate the limitations of virtual media, which is especially important in the hospice and palliative care setting.

The following bullet points offer ways in which the veterinary team can adjust communication practices to better support their clients through difficult end-of-life conversations in a virtual setting:

- To create a greater sense of intimacy, match your "head size" to theirs by positioning your distance to the camera. This most closely mimics an in-person visit.
- Avoid typing or looking at medical records when discussing sensitive or important topics.[5] If you need to refer to medical records or capture an important point, share with the client what you are doing to avoid appearing disinterested or distracted.
- Good eye contact is crucial for increasing personal connection during virtual communication. Remember to look directly at the camera and not the client on the screen. Frequently observe your facial expressions.[6]
- It is important to talk slower on video than you normally would in-person and be sure to check with the client every so often to ensure that you are being heard. If you are having difficulty hearing or understanding, use this opportunity to reinforce connection and trust. Ask, *"What you are saying is really important to me. Can you please repeat what you just shared?"*
- Provide clients with defined pauses to allow them to reflect on, summarize, and repeat information back to you. Pauses also allow the opportunity to assess client understanding and acknowledge their emotions.
- Provide regular reassurance including asking how the client is feeling.

- Display empathy using nonverbal cues and body language. When using body language to convey empathy, make sure it is visible on the client's screen. Physically lean into the camera to show that you are listening. Make sure you are rephrasing what the client says to show that you hear.
- Provide empathetic statements. As facial expressions and body language may be more difficult to interpret via a virtual appointment, members of the hospice team will need to ensure and prioritize empathetic statements so they can respond to a client emotion appropriately.[5] Use phrases such as, "*I can't imagine how difficult this has been for you*" (**Table 1**).
- Allowing the client to express emotions is a critical component of successful palliative and hospice care delivered through telehealth, and it is important to allow space for it. If clients begin to express strong emotions, give them permission to move to a more private setting in the house where they will believe comfortable expressing those emotions. For example, they may not want their children to hear them being upset or if there are other family members present who are not in alignment with their goals or wishes.
- Request the client's permission before discussing a sensitive or difficult topic. Observe verbal and nonverbal responses to gauge whether it is safe to proceed with the conversation.[7] An example would be, "*I understand this is a difficult topic to discuss, but I would like to explain what you can expect during Max's euthanasia. If you are not ready to have this conversation, I understand, and we can revisit this later. Would it be OK to discuss this now, or would you prefer to wait?*"

Table 1 RAVENS: Communication techniques and examples for responding to client emotions	
Techniques	**Examples**
Reflect	"I hear how very sad all of this is for you." "I hear how difficult this is and I wonder if it is even harder right now given that 'Max' belonged to your mom, who also had cancer, and passed away last year?"
Align	"I hear how hard it is to have to think about talking to your children about what all this means. I want you to know that we will be right here with you and will provide the resources needed to help navigate these difficult conversations."
Validate	"I completely understand how difficult it is to live with this uncertainty and not knowing when a decline in 'Max' will happen. It is very scary"
Explore	"When your last pet, 'Sam', was euthanized, what was that experience like for you? Can you share with me more about what the most difficult part was for you and your family?"
Normalize	"You are not alone in feeling this way. Most of my clients believe the same emotions that you are sharing with me. It is so normal to believe anger or guilt that this is happening to 'Max.' It is normal to think, 'if I only would have...,' and I hear this comment from nearly every family that goes through this."
Silence	"....." Moments of silence provide clients with the space needed to process what is being said. The use of nonverbal communication such as empathetic facial expressions or head nodding can help you stay connected to the client during times of silence. The key to knowing when to break the silence is that clients will break the silence themselves first or reengage in eye contact letting you know it is ok to begin speaking again. Silence can believe uncomfortable at times, but it is one of the most powerful communication tools we can use, and veterinary providers should not be afraid to use this technique.

- If a client expresses strong emotions or does not want to continue the conversation, think about how you might want to wind the conversation down. Ending a telehealth session can believe abrupt, and in a virtual setting, we do not get to walk clients to the door or touch their shoulder in a gesture of comfort. An approach in this situation would be to gently move the conversation to a "safer" place so that the client will believe more integrated and less emotional before the visit ends. An example would be, *"We have discussed a lot of emotionally difficult things together today and I understand how hard this can be. If you prefer, we can pause our conversation here and continue it tomorrow; I am here to do whatever feels best for you right now."*
- End-of-life discussions can be just as emotionally draining for the provider as they are for the client. Because of this, it is important to incorporate a "technology time out" in between serial virtual visits to minimize emotional fatigue and to prepare yourself to communicate effectively and be in the moment with your next client.

Techniques for Responding to Client Emotion in a Virtual Setting

Dealing with a client's emotions can believe difficult and uncomfortable, and it can believe even more so in a virtual setting. The following **table 1** illustrates an acronym, "RAVENS," highlighting six techniques that can be used to respond to client emotions along with examples to illustrate possible responses.

FUTURE DIRECTIONS

As a profession, we need to begin to define telehealth-specific end-of-life metrics that focus on delivering the right care at the right time through the right modality, focusing on utilization, compliance, clinical outcomes, cost, and access.

We should simultaneously be generating a more complete evidence base to support telehealth use at end of life. Additional data, including patient, client, and veterinary team experiences; patient outcomes such as symptom management and well-being; and health care utilization, costs, and client compliance are needed to ensure that we are using technology safely and effectively as well as to inform best practices across the field.

Research involving patients who are terminally ill can be difficult because of the perceived vulnerability of the population and professional caution;[8] however, this barrier can be overcome with appropriate communication and client approach, and as clients continue to grow accustomed to receiving care for their pets remotely, there will be more opportunities to engage families in research remotely as well.

SUMMARY

Hospice and palliative care have long been primed for telehealth due to the home-based care design, the access issues inherent for geriatric, ill, or debilitated patients, and the need to reassess end-of-life patients frequently. Telehealth holds great promise for leveraging technology to provide care more effectively and efficiently and is a way to improve and expand the current model of hospice and palliative care.

Although telehealth will not replace all in-person hospice and palliative care visits, it can certainly complement them and a combination of the two methods may be most effective in most circumstances. Telehealth has become not just a beneficial option, but a vital resource, and it has a place in hospice and palliative care as it does in all veterinary health care. As clients continue to learn what is possible and what value they can gain through telehealth for end-of-life care, there will be increasing consumer demand for which veterinary teams will be called on to provide. Telehealth is revolutionizing hospice and palliative care, enhancing the patient–client experience, and easing the many burdens clients are faced with during this challenging time.

Telehospice and telepalliative care are no longer a matter of if, rather, it is now a question of when this level of innovation will become a recognized best practice and what leaders will emerge to help shape the new landscape of care for end-of-life providers.

CLINICS CARE POINTS

Benefits of providing hospice and palliative care via telehealth:
- Increased access: Whenever the veterinary team adds telehealth to their service, patient access increases. Expanded access is especially important for hospice patients as their clinical status can change suddenly.
- Expanded care: Telehealth is not a replacement for the care team but, rather, an expansion. It gives the hospice team more in-depth analysis of the patient's health and allows the hospice team to function more effectively.
- Improved care: Telehealth supports proactive and timely care, improving chronic disease management thereby improving clinical outcomes.
- Improved practice efficiency: Telehealth leverages and supports current staffing, scheduling, and travel times.
- Improved veterinary team experience: Telehealth is a tool to help improve work–life balance, job satisfaction, reduce fatigue and burnout, and staff turnover rate.

PLACES: Key considerations for telehospice and telepalliative care visits:
- *Prepare* with intention
- *Listen* attentively and purposefully
- *Align* with the goals of the client
- *Connect* with the client's story
- *Explore* emotional cues
- *Support* without judgment

DISCLOSURE

The author has no conflicts of interests to declare.

REFERENCES

1. Hiratsuka V, Delafield R, Starks H, et al. Patient and provider perspectives on using telemedicine for chronic disease management among Native Hawaiian and Alaska Native people. Int J Circumpolar Health 2013;72. https://doi.org/10.3402/ijch.v72i0.21401.
2. American Hospital Association Telehealth: Helping Hospitals Deliver Cost Effective Care. AHA. [202028].
3. Steindal S, Nes A, Godskesen T, et al. Patients' Experiences of Telehealth in Palliative Home Care: Scoping Review. J Med Internet Res 2020;22(5):e16218.
4. Al-Quteimat OM, Amer AM. The Impact of the COVID-19 Pandemic on Cancer Patients. Am J Clin Oncol 2020;43(6):452–5.
5. Zulman DM, Haverfield MC, Shaw JG, et al. Practices to Foster Physician Presence and Connection With Patients in the Clinical Encounter. JAMA 2020;323(1):70–81.
6. Ben-Arieh D, Charness N, Duckett K, et al. A Concise Guide for Telemedicine Practitioners: Human Factors Quick Guide Eye Contact. Published February 2016.

7. Flint L, Kotwal A. The New Normal: Key Considerations for Effective Serious Illness Communication Over Video or Telephone During the Coronavirus Disease 2019 (COVID-19) Pandemic. Ann Intern Med 2020;173(6):486–8.

8. Chambers E, Gardiner C, Thompson J, et al. Patient and career involvement in palliative care research: An integrative qualitative evidence synthesis review. Palliat Med 2019;33(8):969–84.

Asynchronous Veterinary Telemedicine

Aaron Smiley, DVM

KEYWORDS

- Telemedicine • Virtual care • VCPR • Remote care • Wearable technology
- Hospice care

KEY POINTS

- Asynchronous communication is an efficient way to offer telemedicine.
- Animal owners are comfortable with asynchronous communication.
- Synchronous and asynchronous communication can be used in tandem.
- A client can be involved in an asynchronous chat between a general practitioner and a board-certified veterinary specialist.

INTRODUCTION

Advancements in technology change the way people communicate. For generations, the telephone was the primary means of remote communication, but now the most common communication in the western world is asynchronous, electronic messaging. Veterinarians can use this cultural shift of communication to improve the efficiency and quality of telemedicine.

Electronic messaging improves the efficiency of telemedicine because it is culturally accepted as an asynchronous communication (ASC). In contrast, a voice conversation requires a continual back-and-forth of information until the call is complete. Pauses in a texting conversation are anticipated and accepted as normal. The acceptance of this asynchronous exchange gives everyone involved in a texting conversation more freedom. A person can engage when it is convenient without frustrating the other people in the conversation.

Finally, asynchronous messaging is the preferred modality of communication for most of the animal owners. Engaging the client through his preferred means of communication lowers barriers of communication between the doctor and client and results in improved care for the patient.

Devonshire Veterinary Clinic, 5030 South Scatterfield, Anderson, IN 46013, USA
E-mail address: aaronsmiley@me.com

Vet Clin Small Anim 52 (2022) 1135–1140
https://doi.org/10.1016/j.cvsm.2022.05.003
0195-5616/22/© 2022 Elsevier Inc. All rights reserved.

DEFINITIONS

Asynchronous communication: Communication that has a variable delay between the sending and receiving of information.

Synchronous communication: Communication that takes place in real time without significant delays between sending and receiving information.

Short Message Service: A technology for sending short text messages between mobile phones. The messages can typically be up to 160 characters in length, though some services use 5 bit mode, which supports 224 characters.

Multimedia Messaging Service: It is a mobile phone service that allows users to send multimedia messages to each other. This includes images, videos, and sound files.

Instant message: A text-based communication similar to chat that uses a shared software client between or among two or more people.

Virtual referral: Telemedicine that involves a board-certified specialist, a generalist and the animal owner.

History of Veterinary Telemedicine

Veterinarians have offered some form of telemedicine since the beginning of modern practice. Before the telephone or telegraph, the doctor could remotely care for patients through written letters to the animal owner. This system was not feasible for most medical problems because of the time it took to have a letter delivered. The long delay between sending and receiving information was fixed with the invention of electronic communication. The telegraph (asynchronous) and later the telephone (synchronous) made communication instantaneous. In addition, the telephone allowed users to experience the modulation of sound. This provided a more nuanced communication to be transmitted, expanding the conditions that could be managed and treated remotely. The animal owner could now hear the veterinarian's voice and glean information from the tone the doctor used to deliver the information to better understand the gravity of the problem. Likewise, the doctor could hear the voice of the owner or the sounds a patient was making and provide better care than if information was only transmitted through the written word. Veterinarians readily adopted the telephone as the vehicle for telemedicine as the technology became ubiquitous in society. Voice calls became so highly integrated into veterinary practice that veterinarians did not even think of it as telemedicine.

The next seismic change in communication occurred with the invention of the Internet. People replaced physical mail with email. This fast ASC matriculated into veterinary telemedicine, but the phone call was still the predominant way the veterinarians offered telemedicine.

In 2007, the first iPhone was released and it married multiple technologies into a handheld unit. The Internet, a QWERTY keyboard, and a quality camera were seamlessly integrated into a single device. Short message service (SMS) messages outnumbered voice calls for the first time in 2010.[1] The default communication shifted from voice calls to SMS messages.

This cultural shift in communication habits and the continual improvement of the smartphone allowed veterinary telemedicine medicine to make a quantum leap forward. Animal owners could now provide high-quality, first-hand data to the doctor in a convenient, asynchronous fashion without any new equipment or training.

Advantages of Asynchronous Communication

ASC is efficient because it does not require the participants to coordinate schedules. A synchronous conversation, even a spontaneous one, requires everyone involved in the exchange to move their attention to the conversation until it is completed. This is not the case for asynchronous exchanges. For example, an email sent during normal business hours to someone on the other side of the world does not disrupt the recipient. He/she will read the email at his/her convenience. However, if that communication was a synchronous exchange, like a voice call, both parties would be required to participate in real time.

Most veterinary telemedicine is not practiced across multiple time zones but asynchronous conversations give all parties more flexibility to exchange information at convenient times. If a veterinarian offers telemedicine inside of an asynchronous conversation, the owner can send the animal's history and pertinent medical images and/ or videos when the animal and owner are available. Likewise, the veterinarian can respond with questions and instructions for the client when time allows. Neither party has to coordinate a premeditated time to engage in remote care.

Although an asynchronous conversation is a highly efficient way to offer telemedicine, synchronous conversations still have a valuable place in remote care. Medical emergencies require the speed of a synchronous conversation, and some sensitive information such as poor test results is best managed via a traditional voice call.

Technology

The speed of change with modern technology is a blessing and a curse for veterinary telemedicine. On the one hand, advancements in technology provide the veterinarian with the ability to manage and treat more conditions, but the doctor must spend mental energy to keep up with the constant changes. For example, the hardware for capturing images has advanced exponentially since the first smartphone. Users can capture cinema quality videos and sound on their mobile device that would have required bags of equipment just 10 years ago. Software advancements are equally stunning. We can now include multiple people across different platforms in asynchronous conversations that contain large data files. This arrangement was unattainable just a few years ago.

Below is a list of capabilities that are readily available to include in telemedicine technology. This list is not meant to endorse any specific company, and the author is not aware of any company that has a technology that includes all of the recommendations. This list is not exhaustive and readers ought to consult with other organizations such as the Veterinary Virtual Care Association for a list of technology recommendations for veterinary telemedicine. It should also be understood that this list will need to be updated as technology advances.

1. Group conversation
    a. The ability to include other veterinarians who are at the same physical practice and/or board-certified specialists to provide a team approach to remote care that will elevate the quality of medicine.
    b. The inclusion of veterinary nurses and technicians in remote care increases efficiencies through client communication, management of care, and the filling of prescriptions.
2. Private messaging inside of a group conversation
    a. Medical professionals are more efficient if they can have private conversations inside of a group conversation that includes the owner.
3. High-resolution videos and images
    a. The number of conditions that can be diagnosed and managed remotely expanded exponentially because clients can send high-quality videos and pictures.

4. Ability to export the SMS conversation as a portable document format or other readable document.
   a. Telemedicine cases are part of the medical record and need to be included in the medical record. Telemedicine technologies do not need to be compatible with the practice's medical record system but telemedicine cases need to be able to be included in the medical record.
5. Payment collection
   a. Veterinarians have offered asynchronous telemedicine for years via email but do not traditionally charge for the service. Collecting payment through the technology that is hosting the case makes the transition from free to paid telemedicine easier.
6. SMS communication for clients
   a. Clients prefer ASC via SMS through native smartphone apps verses apps that have to be downloaded and installed.
7. Allowing medical teams to access telemedicine technology from a desktop computer and a mobile app.
   a. Being able to use the technology on a mobile device and a desktop allows flexibility for the medical team and makes the introduction of a new workflow easier.
8. Privacy and security
   a. Veterinary medical records and the client's personal information need to be kept confidential. This includes security preventing third parties from obtaining the data and/or the technology company sharing personal information.
9. Voice to text capability
   a. Dictating text messages can be an efficient way for doctors and nurses to communicate via SMS. Over the past few years, native dictation software in smartphones has improved immensely to the point that it can learn uncommon medical language without any training.
10. Away message
    a. Telemedicine is unique because it lowers barriers between the veterinarian and the animal owner. This results in better care for the patient but the doctor needs to be able to create healthy boundaries so that his/her work–life balance is maintained. All of the medical professionals using the technology need to be able to turn telemedicine off at their discretion without leaving clients in the lurch. This can be achieved with an automatic away message that is sent when the doctor turns the technology off.

Asynchronous Communication Etiquette

Every form of communication has cultural norms and accepted etiquettes. Asynchronous texting is a newer vehicle for telemedicine, and the best practices for communicating inside of it have not been codified. The list provided is not exhaustive and stems from the author's experience.

1. Emojis
   1. Veterinary telemedicine can be highly emotional because the veterinary team is providing care to animals that are deeply loved by their owners. Emojis allow the care providers to succinctly convey emotion.
   2. Create a library of four to five emojis that represent the most common emotions the veterinary team needs to show to the client.
      1. Specific emojis have different meanings to different cultural groups and can change meaning over time. Include a diverse group of team members when creating the library of acceptable emojis to get a diverse perspective.

3. Emojis can be used as shorthand for intra-office communication. This is beneficial for repeated requests between the doctor and staff such as a request for approval of a prescription.

2. Response time

   1. ASC is efficient because it allows a significant amount of time to lapse between communications but clients need to know what to expect. An expectation for the typical response time of the doctor ought to be communicated to the client at the initiation of the first telemedicine case. This can be achieved via an automatic message generated by the technology or a message from a veterinary team member or the veterinarian himself. Clients become comfortable with delays between messages if they know what to expect. At a minimum, the doctor needs to engage with every telemedicine case once a day. When the nursing team is included in the telemedicine case, the doctor can delegate responsibilities and have the team to collect a history and communicate with the client. The nursing team can also triage patients so the doctor knows what cases need more immediate attention.

3. Shorthand and abbreviations

   1. Texting is typically limited to 160 characters so there is widespread use of abbreviations. The veterinary teams should avoid shorthand when communicating with the owner to avoid misunderstanding. In addition, the veterinary team should get clarification if the owner uses shorthand inside the conversation.

   2. Proper grammar and punctuation should also be maintained to communicate professionalism and communicate clearly.

4. Typos

   1. It is inevitable that typing mistakes will be sent to the client, which need to be corrected. SMS messaging does not allow the sender to edit the message once it is sent, so a mistake can be clarified with an additional message. The author recommends using three asterisks at the start of the message to signal that the following text is a correction of the previous message. For example, if the doctor sends a message to the client, asking for the animal's weight and mistakenly types wait, he should send a second message that begins with *** and then the message.

   2. If the mistake cannot be corrected with a clarifying message, a call is warranted. Someone from the medical team who is involved in the telemedicine case can send a message to the client asking if he/she can call to clarify the message.

Case Selection

Asynchronous telemedicine is not appropriate for every case. The doctor must maintain his/her standard of medical care regardless of how he/she interacts with the client and patient. Some cases are better managed remotely but most require an in-person evaluation. The veterinarian must obtain sufficient information to make an appropriate whether the patient is remote or physically present.

Virtual Referral

Asynchronous telemedicine is a convenient way to involve the client in a conversation between the general practitioner and the veterinary specialist. In the past, the general practitioner would either refer a case or consult with the specialist. Now, asynchronous telemedicine allows the client to enter the conversation and engage directly with the veterinary specialist.

The American Veterinary Medical Association (AVMA)/American Animal Hospital Assocation (AAHA) 2021 Telehealth Guidelines for Small-Animal Practice endorse a three-way conversation between the generalist, the specialist, and the client. This arrangement is a newer way to refer veterinary patients and increases access to care, but cannot be used for every case. Both the generalist and the specialist will use their medical expertise to determine if the case is eligible for virtual referral (VR). VR simplifies the referral process because the specialist can ask specific questions to the generalist and the client in lieu of lengthy or incomplete referral forms. It also minimizes the wait time to see a specialist. Clients can start a consultation within days instead of weeks, and they do not have to travel to a new clinic.

In addition, VR reduces the burden on the veterinary emergency clinic because clients are less likely to present nonemergencies through the emergency room just to gain access to the veterinary specialist. The three stakeholders enter into an asynchronous texting conversation. Medical information (images and videos), history, and test results are provided by the general practitioner and the client, and care is provided through the general practitioner.

To the author's best knowledge, the legal ramifications of VR have not been published outside of this article. The AVMA/AHHA published guidelines for telemedicine in 2020 and endorsed a three-way conversation between the general practitioner, the specialist, and the client. It is assumed that the general practitioner holds the liability for the medical case because he/she holds the Veteirnary Client Patient Relationship (VCPR). All veterinarians involved have the burden to practice according the standards of the profession.

SUMMARY

ASC is an efficient way for the veterinarian to offer high-quality remote care. Clients prefer communicating via asynchronous texting on native smartphone apps. Veterinary nurses and technicians can provide medical and customer support for telemedicine cases, similarly to the support they offer in the physical clinic. Last, a board-certified veterinary specialist can engage directly with the client if the general practitioner is included in a three-way conversation.

DISCLOSURE

A. Smiley is Chief Veterinarian at Medici, a human health company, and provides telemedicine to his clients in central Indiana as a Chief of Staff for VetCor.

REFERENCE

1. Gayomali C. The text message turns 20: a brief history of SMS. The Week 2015.

Small Animal Teleultrasound

Timothy Manzi, VMD, DACVR, DACVR-EDI*,
Cristobal Navas de Solis, LV, PhD, DACVIM (LA)

KEYWORDS

- Teleultrasound • Telesonography • Ultrasound • Teleradiology • Telemedicine

KEY POINTS

- Teleultrasound is becoming a prominent form of telemedicine in the veterinary profession as access to ultrasound to the general practitioner increases at a greater rate compared with the number of imaging specialists.
- Two main methods of teleultrasound currently exist: asynchronous and synchronous interpretations.
- No standardized protocols for small animal teleultrasound are available.
- Factors affecting the success of a telesonographic interpretation are the technological aspects, the quality of the acquired images, the quality of the interpretation, and the relationship between the on-site veterinarian and the imaging expert.

INTRODUCTION

Telemedicine and particularly teleradiology have become a prominent feature of veterinary medicine within the last 25 years but this health-care tool has been around for more than a century.[1] Teleradiology developed throughout the 1900s as technology and medical imaging devices improved and became more refined. In recent years, the use of teleultrasound—or the remote interpretation of an ultrasound study—in human medicine has been more common in cardiology, obstetrics, and POCUS. However, ultrasound has a very steep learning curve in both acquisition and interpretation and is considered the most operator-dependent of all imaging modalities.[2]

In veterinary medicine, both the interest and availability of ultrasound machines to general practitioners in many areas has outpaced both the ultrasound training provided in veterinary schools and the number of imaging specialists to interpret these studies. Clinician performed ultrasounds are common in veterinary medicine and are likely to increase in number, following trends in human medicine.[3] Training programs in the university and continuing education setting are likely to progressively

University of Pennsylvania, Clinical Studies New Bolton Center, 382 West Street Road, Kennett Square, PA 19348, USA
* Corresponding author.
E-mail address: timmanzi@vet.upenn.edu

Vet Clin Small Anim 52 (2022) 1141–1151
https://doi.org/10.1016/j.cvsm.2022.05.004
0195-5616/22/Published by Elsevier Inc.

vetsmall.theclinics.com

fill current gaps. The application of teleultrasound in human medicine has proven to be highly effective, and the rapid access to imaging experts by sonographers at the patient's side can have a positive impact on patient care.[4,5] Currently, many veterinary practices do not have direct access to an imaging specialist, and this is unlikely to soon change. Radiologists or imaging experts at a different location from where images are acquired (eg, teleradiologists) are likely to be essential to provide the best medical care possible.

Teleradiologists have been a feature of small animal veterinary practices in more recent years, as a surrogate for the "in-person" radiologist. This has historically been the most used form of telehealth in veterinary medicine but, in general, there has been less emphasis placed on developing teleultrasound than other imaging modalities.[6] With a vast landscape before it, teleultrasound has a substantial opportunity for growth within the veterinary profession and is likely to greatly enhance the armamentarium of the general veterinary practitioner, although it is not without its own technological and logistical peculiarities and even few impediments.

TECHNICAL ASPECTS

Initially in the 1990s, when teleradiology was first becoming a feature of veterinary practices, large file sizes and slow connection speeds were often insurmountable barriers. These problems have since largely been resolved and virtual access to imaging specialists around the world currently requires infrastructure that is often already present in most veterinary practices in western societies. Teleradiology in limited resource or rural settings with limited Internet connectivity and access to information technology expertise is inherently more difficult.

The teleradiology guidelines from the American College of Veterinary Radiology (ACVR)[7] focus on the type of files (eg, Digital Imaging and Communications in Medicine (DICOM)), aspects of image compression, and file transfer. The guidelines mainly refer to "store-and-forward" transmissions and do not specifically mention ultrasound. For the transmission of store-and-forward ultrasound studies, there are similar logistics as what currently exist for the transmission of images of other modalities, although there is the additional factor to consider that analyzing large cine loops is a frequent need. For real-time teleultrasound, the image quality and degradation through transmission can be significant barriers to successful implementation.[2] Studies in the 1990s showed that the quality of dynamic ultrasound images transmitted at 384 kbit/s was diagnostically acceptable but unsatisfactory at 128 kbit/s, and that diagnostic accuracy for remote fetal ultrasound studies was marginally worse at the lower bandwidth (384 kbit/s vs 1920 kbit/s).[8] Other studies have suggested that 600 kbit/s and 30 frames per second (fps) is the threshold for the maintenance of diagnostic image quality.[9] For reference, common frame rates for teleconference systems are 15 to 30 fps. Typical 4G mobile networks may have upload speeds between 2 and 50 Mbits/s, whereas most domestic connections exceed this. 5G networks will likely soon increase the speed of connection to the hundreds of Mbit/s or exceed a Gbit/s.

Anecdotally, the authors have found that "Internet speed tests" are often not reliable to determine if the quality of a live ultrasound will be sufficient. Therefore, the authors prefer to perform a trial with the equipment and location that will be used. Nevertheless, a very low speed can be a limiting factor. In the authors' setting, the 600 kbit/s mentioned in the literature typically will establish communication, and 1 Mbit/s upload speed is likely to provide a teleconference that includes one video feed without disruptions. An Internet connection with 2 to 5 Mbits/s upload speed and 15 to 20 Mbit/s download speed is very likely to support adequate connections with 2 simultaneous video feeds and 2-way verbal communication. The specific ultrasound device, video processing, image capture device, computer/tablet used to emit and receive, teleconference software, video settings of the software, download speed or latency are also factors that play a role in the transmission. It is also important to note that in many situations, bandwidth is shared between different devices, and this can play a role in the variation of quality at a given time. Additionally, security of the Internet connections and transmissions when using teleultrasound is an important consideration that needs to be managed analogously to other cybersecurity concerns of the veterinary practice.

Asynchronous, or "store-and-forward," telemedicine involves collecting information that is later forwarded to an expert for interpretation. Asynchronous assistance is performed at a larger scale by most teleradiology companies but fewer companies offer synchronous assistance in veterinary ultrasound. Most ultrasound equipment and software allow for nearly instantaneous upload and sharing of images on different formats, including DICOM. Images and clips are stored most frequently but audio and text can also potentially be transmitted. This mode eliminates the need to coordinate the schedule of the remote expert, the individual acquiring images, and the patient. This is widely used when technicians or trainees perform ultrasounds and is likely the most widespread mode of teleultrasound. The biggest disadvantage is the inability of the remote expert to control that image quality, type of images, and patient information.[10]

In contrast, synchronous telemedicine refers to a communication in which the on-site and remote veterinarian occurs in real-time. This type of communication often implies mirroring/sharing the screen of the ultrasound equipment or using embedded software in the ultrasound equipment that allows the remote expert to see the image as it is being acquired. This allows the remote expert to be part of the interpretation and the image acquisition process. It has been noted that the on-site veterinarians often perceive this process as a learning activity. Importantly, this system may allow earlier detection of problems in acquisition of images or gathering of patient information, and animal owners have reported positive experiences and think a higher level of care is provided to their animals when this modality is used.[10–13] Sonograms performed with remote assistance have been reported to be longer than sonograms performed by an expert or a nonexpert without assistance even when not accounting for time spent coordinating schedules of individuals involved. The authors are unaware of a direct comparison between synchronous and asynchronous telemedicine for ultrasound. It is intuitive that the real-time assistance provides potentially more beneficial components to communications, mentoring, and imaging acquisition processes, whereas technical and logistical issues may affect the speed and efficiency but this impression would need to be proven.[1]

Some portable and ultraportable ultrasound equipment have embedded software that allows sharing the ultrasound image, a live image of the patient screen and a 2-way verbal communication making real-time telemedicine easier to organize. In some setups, the remote expert can control the ultrasound machine remotely. Most standard teleconference systems and telemedicine applications allow 1 or 2 simultaneous video feeds, and the image from an ultrasound device can often be fed into the teleconference software connecting the ultrasound device to a computer or tablet. Most current teleconference software also allows storage of video that can be reviewed or become part of the medical record. This should not substitute saving images in high quality (eg, DICOM) formats. There are telemedicine companies that provide the infrastructure, equipment, training, and assistance with acquisition and interpretation of images. Low-cost solutions to establish connections to perform teleultrasound are feasible with an end result of a standard teleconference in which the video input is the real-time sonogram. This can be achieved using off-the-shelf software and hardware including the existing ultrasound equipment. This is achieved by connecting the video port of the ultrasound device (often using High-Definition multimedia interface (HDMI), Digital visual interface (DVI), Video graphics array (VGA) cable) to a capture devices/video converters (such as Epiphan AV.io HD Video Grabber, Palo Alto, California, USA) and then to a computer or tablet that is using videoconference software.[14–16] The goals, ability to streamline, and cost-effectiveness differences will dictate the most adequate solution for each individual situation.

TRAINING AND EDUCATION

The skill and knowledge of the sonographer acquiring images is a rate-limiting step to the quality of images and completeness of studies. This can significantly affect diagnostic accuracy, add time and financial costs to the veterinary practice, and ultimately affect patient care.[2,10] Training to obtain and interpret ultrasound images is as—if not more—important to teleultrasound as it is to on-site ultrasounds.

In a recent review of teleultrasound for humans, one study stated that "...in small medical centers, untrained operators could not capture appropriate ultrasound views, even with real-time vocal guidance."[17] Another study showed that real-time teleultrasound including verbal communication could overcome the lack of trained operators in remote or underdeveloped regions.[18] In a recent publication, tele-intensivists guided nonphysicians with minimal ultrasound training to acquire clinically useful images without compromising quality between images saved directly from the ultrasound and those viewed with a camera in the ICU.[19] The investigators suggested that training medical personnel (clinical practitioners, residents, and nonintensivist physicians) and using the critical care ultrasound-trained physician to enhance POCUS training via tele-ICU would be a positive addition to the ICU workflow. These and other studies[20] may indicate that teleultrasound is a heterogeneous and multifactorial process. It is likely that not all operators can be guided by any expert to perform all types of ultrasounds. Furthermore, a single answer to the question *"Is teleultrasound a possible and beneficial tool?"* may not exist and factors that include personnel, indication, logistics, equipment can easily tilt the balance negatively.

In some situations, there is a disparity between practitioner's access to ultrasound and expertise.[21] Veterinary curricula are changing to provide training in ultrasound image acquisition and interpretation, but currently advanced training is reserved to diagnostic imaging residencies. In North America, these residencies are under the purview of the ACVR. The ACVR has noted that diagnostic ultrasound is one of the most frequently requested imaging tests ordered for small animal patients, although the results of the examination can either be hindered or facilitated by the skill of the sonographer.[22] Although in human medicine it is common and proven that diagnostic ultrasound images can be acquired by nonphysician if overseen by a physician, this is a less common scenario in veterinary medicine.[1,20,21]

Few veterinary diagnostic imaging residencies have a formal—or even informal—component of telemedicine built into their training, despite greater than one-third of board-certified radiologists incorporating some degree of teleradiology into their daily practice.[23] Similarly, there is also no uniform training or protocols for nonspecialists to learn how to acquire a diagnostic sonographic study consistently and effectively if it is to be sent to an imaging specialist for interpretation. Although teleradiology and other veterinary companies have courses designed to teach veterinarians the basics in small animal ultrasound acquisition and interpretation, standardization between them is rare. Training via teleultrasound[24–26] has been shown to be feasible, have a high user satisfaction, and train sonographers with good diagnostic accuracy when compared with on-site training. Both synchronous and asynchronous teleultrasound teaching methods have been shown to be potentially effective.[26] A recent study of focused cardiac ultrasound telesupervised physicians performed scans of better quality than nonsupervised physicians, supporting the use of telesupervision for physicians with basic focused US competence.[15] All this information suggests that imaging experts being involved in study acquisition can benefit the diagnostic process. Teleultrasound and the virtual setting provides new logistic opportunities for teaching that may help the veterinary profession increase accessibility and quality of training in addition to its diagnostic capabilities.[20]

Veterinary education is evolving, and traditional models based on a curriculum that relies heavily on classroom teaching are being challenged. Telementoring has been proven to be an adequate means of medical education on the patient side,[27] and the logistical advantages of remote and self-driven learning[28] have been highlighted during the COVID-19 pandemic. Ultrasound has been proposed to be important in clinical and preclinical medical curricula not only as an imaging modality but also as a tool to engage students in active learning and provide better understanding of core disciplines such as anatomy or physiology. There are many unknowns and controversies about what role ultrasound should play in education[29] and the best strategies to combine in person and remote education tools. The discussion will continue in years to come as veterinary schools undergo curriculum redesign and teleultrasound deserves a seat at the table.[30]

PROTOCOLS

There are no widely established or standardized protocols for veterinary teleultrasound. Most telemedicine companies provide guidance about format and information to submit in studies. The ACVR position statement on ultrasound[22] defines minimum expectations for a competent veterinary sonographer during the acquisition and interpretation of sonographic studies but no specific guidelines regarding images that should be acquired or recommendations regarding technological aspects of image acquisition are specified. In contrast, human medicine counterparts (American College of Radiology) have generated a litany of documents on a range of teleradiology/teleultrasound such as licensure and legal requirements, international limitations, or technology recommendations.[31,32]

Telemedicine companies offering teleultrasound have taken different approaches to logistics. A few examples are used here for readers' information, whereas other companies may have a different approach with a similar value. For example, one large veterinary telemedicine company has compiled a list of images/cine loops, file sizes, formats, and duration of clips required for submission.[33] This follows the ACVR proposed concept[22] that for this type of asynchronous submission to be effective, the individual performing the ultrasound study must possess a thorough understanding of the normal and abnormal sonographic appearance of the structures being examined and be able to accurately acquire all the required images/cine loops. Another large teleradiology company provides no specific list or rigid guidelines regarding file size and the numbers of images that may be submitted. This company opts for providing the submitter virtual access to a radiologist to facilitate communication and hopefully enhance diagnostic value. This company also requests that the submitter includes impressions of the study to help better inform the teleradiologist.[34] Other companies have opted for assuming responsibility for more aspects of the interaction including providing uniform ultrasound equipment that can be controlled remotely, train the sonographer acquiring images, provide real-time support during the acquisition of images, and provide specialist interpretation of the images.[35] There are no veterinary studies comparing diagnostic accuracy, efficiency, or indications for the different solutions. Although it is likely that "real-time" image acquisition provides more information and that cine loop(s) provide more information than a singular static image, the time invested is likely directly proportional to the information obtained. More time-consuming processes may be less efficient or feasible in some clinical scenarios or business models but perhaps needed in others. Prospective studies in different scenarios and indications would be needed to prove these clinical impressions.

A predetermined checklist of representative images and cine loops can minimize the loss of relevant information. The authors provide here an example of a list of recommended images and information to include when submitting a telesonographic study of the small animal abdomen. Of significant note is that the information provided in **Box 1** is based on personal experience and merged with other resources available and therefore inherently subjective. The intent is to provide *minimum* standards for what images should be included, balancing efficiency, and diagnostic yield. This information is *not* meant to be applied to all clinical situations but perhaps provides a starting framework for teleultrasound studies that should be tested prospectively. Independent of the platform, company, or tools, consistency between studies is important. In addition to the expertise of the professional obtaining images and the expertise of professional interpreting images, the interaction between the 2 is a critical but difficult to define or quantify factor. Nonetheless, it is clear these factors can be linked to the efficiency and the quality of the reporting.

DIAGNOSTIC ACCURACY

To the best of our knowledge, there are no peer-reviewed publications evaluating the diagnostic accuracy of teleultrasound in veterinary medicine. A recent study in horses reported the feasibility of performing synchronous teleultrasound. In 40% of the interactions, the sonogram was perceived as useful for clinical management. In 40%, reassurance to veterinarians or owners was the reported main value and in 20% of the cases educational value was considered the most important aspect of the interaction.[11]

Studies in human medicine may help us gain some insights until more veterinary studies are performed, and the topic has been recently reviewed.[2] For example, the diagnostic accuracy of teleultrasound for the detection of birth defects in humans was analogous to the accuracy for on-site ultrasound.[36] POCUS performed by pediatricians and guided remotely by expert radiologists had high accuracy (sensitivity, specificity, positive and negative predictive values of 88.2%, 99.7%, 96.8%, 98.7%, respectively) when compared with radiologist on site and agreement between pediatricians and the radiologist was excellent (k = 0.93).[4] A study testing the diagnostic accuracy of cardiac, abdominal, and thoracic POCUS in an ICU showed 100% concordance in the image interpretation by the on-site intensivist and tele-ICU physicians. When the recorded video clips were reviewed by the third blinded intensivist, concordance regarding study results was also 100%. In this scenario, the diagnostic accuracy of on-site veterinarian, real-time remote assessment and store and forward assessment was equal.[37] In a study in which paramedics performed lung POCUS of the lungs in patients with respiratory distress[38] and images were interpreted asynchronously by experts in ultrasound 25% of scans could not be completed due to equipment failure, 58.8% of completed scans were deemed uninterpretable and the agreement between emergency medical services physicians and experts was poor.

Box 1
Technical/general information

- Sonographer contact information
  - Name
  - Phone number
  - E-mail address
- Patient's first and last name
- Signalment
- Date of study
- Number of images/cine loops submitted
- Relevant history
- Clinical questions to be answered
- Brief ultrasound findings/interpretation

Recommended Images/Cine Loops:
  Small animal abdominal ultrasound

At least 2 orthogonal (eg, at ~90° perpendicular to each other) static images of each of the following should be included, with additional images and cine loops of areas relevant to clinical questions or with suspected sonographic pathologic condition to be included at the discretion of the sonographer.

- Kidneys
  - Renal pelvis
  - Ureters *(as much as can be imaged)*
- Liver
  - Left, right, and central divisions
- Gall bladder
  - Biliary tree *(as much as can be imaged)*
  - Major duodenal papilla
- Spleen
  - Splenic vein hilus
- Urinary Bladder
  - Trigone/ureterovesicular junctions
- Sublumbar/retroperitoneal space
  - Medial iliac lymph nodes
  - Aorta
  - Caudal vena cava
- Pancreas/region of the pancreas
  - Right lobe/body *(typically more commonly identified in dogs)*
  - Left lobe *(typically more commonly identified in cats)*
- Adrenal Glands
- Stomach
  - Cardia *(if possible)*
  - Pylorus
- Small Intestines
- Colon
  - Ileocolic junction
    - More commonly seen in cats and may be seen in dogs
- Mesenteric lymph nodes
- Reproductive tract *(as applicable)*

- ○ Uterus/uterine stump
- ○ Uterine horns
- ○ Ovaries
- ○ Prostate
- ○ Testicles

The use of teleultrasound in that scenario did not meet the criteria they had determined for implementation. Literature suggests that the diagnostic accuracy of on-site and remote radiologists in selected clinical scenarios is analogous if high quality standards for protocols, equipment, image quality, and communication are maintained but accuracy is low in some other situations.In these studies, mentioned benefits of teleultrasound include a quicker time to diagnosis and the ability to provide care in circumstances where expertise or resources would be otherwise limited.[10] This impression may need to be tested in different veterinary situations.

ARTIFICIAL INTELLIGENCE

Although largely beyond the scope of this article, the topic of artificial intelligence (AI), or the application of computer-generated algorithms to perform tasks without the need of human input, has recently garnered significant attention in the world of veterinary imaging and is interrelated with telehealth. Although still in its infancy, the idea that AI may be able to give an accurate interpretation of an imaging study in a location where there is otherwise no access to a radiologist and/or to improve radiologists' efficiency, accuracy, and patient outcomes is desirable for some[39] and feared by others. To the best of the authors' knowledge, the use of AI in the field of veterinary sonography is currently nonexistent.

In contrast, human medicine has explored AI teleultrasound. Studies on this topic include the ability of a completely teleoperated system consisting of a robotic arm[40] or motorized transducers[41] to change settings remotely. These studies have shown that these devices were able to obtain adequate images in 97% of cases of miscellaneous body parts in an area isolated from trained sonographers. Even still, literature specifically regarding the use of AI in sonography is limited, likely due to the highly operator dependent and nuanced way these studies are acquired.

There are also legal, ethical, social, and logistical concerns regarding incorporating AI into veterinary medicine. An expert panel report regarding the use of AI from the ACVR makes no mention of ultrasound and specifically states that the direction of further application of use of AI in veterinary diagnostic imaging is focused on radiology of the thorax in dogs and cats. Although unproven and unstudied, AI in veterinary medicine may initially become more prominent in areas of more straightforward pattern recognition and provide quality assurance of studies that are to be ultimately interpreted by a teleradiologist.[42] Regardless of the ultimate use, imaging specialists will need to guide this complicated endeavor and the wide use of AI in sonography seems unlikely in the near future. What the future holds for the relationship between AI and imaging would be a good topic for an editorial beyond the scope of this article.

SUMMARY

There are many factors that play a role in the success of teleultrasound. Technology, training protocols, clinical information available, equipment, medical indication, communication, the relationship between the on-site and remote veterinarians, and the interactions among all these factors are likely relevant. Teleultrasound is feasible and well received by most animal owners, practitioners, specialty trainees, and sonography experts, and the existing technological challenges can, most of the time, be solved. Addition of clinically useful information, expanding care in remote areas, reassurance to practitioners and animal owners and education for practitioners are all potential benefits of teleultrasound. There are suggestions to support that teleultrasound can increase the quality of veterinary medicine in the future and if implemented wisely, improve animal health, client satisfaction, the quality of veterinary care and provide new opportunities for learning and collaboration worldwide.[11] Ultimately, the creation of knowledge and prioritizing animal health, animal welfare, and the veterinary profession should guide future decisions regarding the incorporation of teleultrasound into daily practice.

CLINICS CARE POINTS

- Teleultrasound is likely to become more commonplace in the clinical work-up in veterinary species in the coming years.
- The 2 main methods of submitting a telesonography study to a teleradiologist include "store-and-forward"/asynchronous and real-time/synchronous.
- A standardized protocol and set of images and cine loops to include when submitting an ultrasound examination to be interpreted by a teleradiologist does not exist but should be pre-established between the individual acquiring the images and the individual ultimately providing the interpretation of the study.
- Factors affecting the success of a telesonographic interpretation are the technological aspects, the quality of the acquired images, the quality of the interpretation, and the relationship between the on-site veterinarian and the imaging expert.

CONFLICT OF INTEREST

The authors have no relevant conflicts of interest to disclose.

REFERENCES

1. Britton N, Miller MA, Safadi S, et al. Tele-Ultrasound in Resource-Limited Settings: A Systematic Review. Front Public Health 2019;7:244.
2. Ferreira AC, O'Mahony E, Oliani AH, et al. Teleultrasound: historical perspective and clinical application. Int J Telemed Appl 2015;2015:306259.
3. Baston CM, Wallace P, Chan W, et al. Innovation Through Collaboration: Creation of a Combined Emergency and Internal Medicine Point-of-Care Ultrasound Fellowship. J Ultrasound Med 2019;38:2209–15.
4. Zennaro F, Neri E, Nappi F, et al. Real-Time Tele-Mentored Low Cost "Point-of-Care US" in the Hands of Paediatricians in the Emergency Department: Diagnostic Accuracy Compared to Expert Radiologists. PLoS One 2016;11(10): e0164539.
5. Salerno A, Tupchong K, Verceles AC, et al. Point-of-Care Teleultrasound: A Systematic Review. Telemed J E Health 2020;26:1314–21.
6. Poteet BA. Veterinary teleradiology. Vet Radiol Ultrasound 2008;49:S33–6.
7. ACVR Teleradiology Guidelines. Available at: https://acvr.org/how-we-do-it/types-of-imaging-therapy/radiology/teleradiology-guidelines/. Accessed January 21, 2022.

8. Wootton R, Dornan J, Fisk NM, et al. The effect of transmission bandwidth on diagnostic accuracy in remote fetal ultrasound scanning. J Telemed Telecare 1997;3:209–14.

9. Yoo SK, Kim DK, Jung SM, et al. Performance of a web-based, realtime, tele-ultrasound consultation system over high-speed commercial telecommunication lines. J Telemed Telecare 2004;10:175–9.

10. Papageorges M, Hebert P, Hanson J, et al. Telesonography. Clin Tech Small Anim Pract 2001;16:117–21.

11. Navas de Solis C, Bevevino K, Doering A, et al. Real-time telehealth using ultrasonography is feasible in equine practice. Equine Vet Educ 2020;32:218–22.

12. Lanevschi-Pietersma A, Boroffka S, Martinez-Pereira Y, et al. Telemedicine: a time management and learning tool for vets and service clinics and what it can offer to pet owners. Eur J Companion Anim Pract 2011;21:73–6.

13. Teller LM, Moberly HK. Veterinary telemedicine: a literature review. Vet Evid 2020;5(4).

14. Adambounou K, Adjenou V, Salam AP, et al. A low-cost tele-imaging platform for developing countries. Front Public Health 2014;2:135.

15. Jensen SH, Weile J, Aagaard R, et al. Remote real-time supervision via tele-ultrasound in focused cardiac ultrasound: A single-blinded cluster randomized controlled trial. Acta Anaesthesiol Scand 2019;63:403–9.

16. Pang DSJ, Pang JM, Payne OJ, et al. Teleconsulting in the time of a global pandemic: Application to anesthesia and technological considerations. Can Vet J 2020;61:1092–100.

17. Adambounou K, Farin F, Boucher A, et al. System of telesonography with synchronous teleconsultations and asynchronus telediagnosis. Med Sante Trop 2012;22:54–60.

18. Popov V, Popov D, Kacar I, et al. The feasibility of realtime transmission of sonographic images from a remote location over low bandwith Internet links: a pilot study. AJR Am J Roentgenol 2007;188:219–22.

19. Levine AR, McCurdy MT, Zubrow MT, et al. Tele-intensivists can instruct non-physicians to acquire high-quality ultrasound images. J Crit Care 2015;30:871–5.

20. Constantinescu EC, Nicolau C, Săftoiu A. Recent Developments in Tele-Ultrasonography. Curr Health Sci J 2018;44:101–6.

21. Becker C, Fusaro M, Patel D, et al. The Utility of Teleultrasound to Guide Acute Patient Management. Cardiol Rev 2017;25:97–101.

22. American College of Veterinary Radiology (ACVR): Position Statement on Ultrasound. Available at: https://acvr.org/how-we-do-it/types-of-imaging-therapy/ultrasound/position-statement-on-ultrasound-by-the-acvr/. Accessed January 21, 2021.

23. Fischetti AJ, Shiroma JT, Poteet BA. Academic and private practice partnerships in veterinary radiology residency training. Vet Radiol Ultrasound 2017;58:367–72.

24. Smith A, Addison R, Rogers P, et al. Remote mentoring of point-of-care ultrasound skills to inexperienced operators using multiple telemedicine platforms: is a cell phone good enough? J Ultrasound Med 2018;37:2517–25.

25. Arntfield RT. The utility of remote supervision with feedback as a method to deliver high-volume critical care ultrasound training. J Crit Care 2015;30:441.

26. Lipsitz M, Levin L, Sharma V, et al. The State of Point-of-Care Teleultrasound Use for Educational Purposes: A Scoping Review. J Ultrasound Med 2021;26. https://doi.org/10.1002/jum.15885.

27. Russell PM, Mallin M, Youngquist ST, et al. First "glass" education: telementored cardiac ultrasonography using Google Glass- a pilot study. Acad Emerg Med 2014;21:1297–9.

28. Williams ZJ, Sage A, Valberg SJ. Hand-Held Point-of-Care Ultrasound: A New Tool for Veterinary Student Self-Driven Learning in the time of COVID-19. J Vet Med Educ 2021;10:e20200131.

29. Davis JJ, Wessner CE, Potts J, et al. Ultrasonography in Undergraduate Medical Education: A Systematic Review. J Ultrasound Med 2018;37:2667–79.

30. Chaney KP, Macik ML, Turner JS, et al. Curriculum Redesign in Veterinary Medicine: Part I. J Vet Med Educ 2017;44(3):552–62.

31. Silva E III, Breslau J, Barr RM, et al. ACR white paper on teleradiology practice: a report from the Task Force on Teleradiology Practice. J Am Coll Radiol 2013;10: 575–85.

32. ACR-AAPM-SIIM Technical Standard for Electronic Practice of Medical Imaging. Available at: https://siim.org/page/practice_guidelines. Accessed January 21, 2022.

33. IDEXX Abdominal Ultrasound Checklist Telemedicine. Available at: https://www. idexx.com/files/abdominal-ultrasound-checklist-telemedicine.pdf.   Accessed January 21, 2022.

34. Antech   ultrasound   reporting   guidelines.   Available   at: https:// antechimagingservices.com/antechweb/ultrasound.   Accessed   January   21, 2022.

35. Real Time Video Assisted Ultrasounds. Oncura Partners. Available at. https:// www.oncurapartners.com/. Accessed January 31, 2022.

36. Rabie NZ, Sandlin AT, Barber KA, et al. Teleultrasound: How Accurate Are We? J Ultrasound Med 2017;36:2329–35.

37. Zaidi G, Dhar S, Chen L, et al. Accuracy of interpretation of point of care ultrasound images in critically ill patients via telemedicine. Chest 2015; 148(4_MeetingAbstracts):331A.

38. Becker TK, Martin-Gill C, Callaway CW, et al. Feasibility of Paramedic Performed Prehospital Lung Ultrasound in Medical Patients with Respiratory Distress. Prehosp Emerg Care 2018;22:175–9.

39. Owens JM, Lewis R, Blevins W, et al. Veterinary radiology-history, purpose, current status and future expectations. Lett Vet Radiol Ultrasound 2019;60:358–62.

40. Georgescu M, Sacccomandi A, Baudron B, et al. Remote Sonography in Routine Clinical Practice Between Two Isolated Medical Centers and the University Hospital Using a Robotic Arm: A 1-Year Study. Telemed J E Health 2016;22:276–81.

41. Arbeille P, Provost R, Zuj K, et al. Teles-operated echocardiography using a robotic arm and an internet connection. Ultrasound Med Biol 2014;40(10):2521–9.

42. American College of Veterinary Radiology (ACVR) statement on Artificial Intelligence in Veterinary Diagnostic Imaging and Radiation Oncology. Available at: https://acvr.org/artificial-intelligence-in-veterinary-diagnostic-imaging-and-radiation-oncology/. Accessed January 21, 2022.

Moving?

Make sure your subscription moves with you!

To notify us of your new address, find your **Clinics Account Number** (located on your mailing label above your name), and contact customer service at:

Email: journalscustomerservice-usa@elsevier.com

800-654-2452 (subscribers in the U.S. & Canada)
314-447-8871 (subscribers outside of the U.S. & Canada)

Fax number: 314-447-8029

Elsevier Health Sciences Division
Subscription Customer Service
3251 Riverport Lane
Maryland Heights, MO 63043

*To ensure uninterrupted delivery of your subscription, please notify us at least 4 weeks in advance of move.

Printed and bound by CPI Group (UK) Ltd, Croydon, CR0 4YY

13/10/2024

01773502-0001